Confessions
OF A CANCER
CONQUEROR

FREE Bonus Material to give you a head start

This book includes

- a Video Book Guide of the main chapters
- Practical cheat sheets
- a Special time- and money saving Gift for you

to allow you to start transforming your relationship with cancer right away.

Get it right here at

http://www.kirstinscancercare.com/ awesomebookbonuses/

ENDORSEMENTS

Dr. Heather Paulson, ND, FABNO: As a naturopathic oncologist, I love the way Kirstin breaks down the fads and trends of cancer diets into something easy and applicable to everyone! She has such gift for seeing what needs to be talked about, and providing the tools to make the changes that could actually help prevent cancer. I can't wait to have my patients read this book.

Dr. Heather Paulson, ND, FABNO, Owner of *The Paulson Center for Integrative Healing* and author of the soon to be released *"Textbook of Naturopathic Oncology"*.

Dr. Evan Hirsch, MD, ABOIM: Kirstin's perspective on our relationship to cancer is refreshing. Using cancer as a vehicle for transformation is exactly how it should be viewed. This is the healthiest way of dealing with cancer. As a physician, I see the emotions of cancer regularly and find that those people who are most successful in their cancer journeys are the ones that transform their minds while they are treating their bodies. Working with Kirstin is a gift.

Evan Hirsch, MD, ABOIM, bestselling author of *"Fix Your Fatigue: The Four Step Process to Resolving Chronic Fatigue, Achieving Abundant Energy and Reclaiming Your Life!"*

Sarica Cernohous, L.Ac., MSTOM, BSBA: Every one of us has been touched by cancer—either as a personal diagnosis and journey of body and soul, or as a diagnosis of a close relation -possibly a family member, a dear friend, a co-worker, a teacher—to be alive in the 21st Century is to know cancer in some way. It is in such an experience we can find ourselves feeling a range of emotions—shock, anger, fear, numbness, sadness.

Kirstin's generous and loving insight and support is the very essence of clarity in this often murky ordeal. With care, she holds our hand as we look at our lifestyle choices and how simple changes can have a profound impact on our wellness, helping us to move from the reactions of shock and fear to a creative expression of hope and empowerment; this is a gift of love that allows us to put into play actionable, simple and powerful steps in the wake of a cancer diagnosis.

Sarica Cernohous, L.Ac., MSTOM, BSBA, bestselling author of *"The Funky Kitchen! The Missing Link in Your Nutrition and Wellness."*

Kerry McClure, BS, RYT, NC, BCHN: "Confessions Of A Cancer Conqueror" is a beautiful compilation of Kirstin's own personal journey with cancer, hope, science and empowering possibilities. Each cancer journey is unique. Kirstin's passion for nutrition and wellness shines through in her mindful writing of this book as a guide to inform and support you in choosing what will be the right healing path for you. This is an important resource for all cancer patients.

Kerry McClure, *BS, RYT, NC, BCHN, Co-Author of "Beyond Meditation: making mindfulness accessible for everyone".*

Mira Dessey, NE: Born out of a personal journey and fueled by a desire to support and encourage others, Kirstin Nussgruber clearly and intelligently delivers an information-packed book on reducing your toxic burden with holistic strategies for food and environmental concerns, as well as addressing physical, and emotional needs. If you or someone you love is concerned about cancer this book is one you should definitely read.

Mira Dessey, NE, The Ingredient Guru and author of *"The Pantry Principle: How to Read the Label and Understand What's Really in your Food"*.

Pat Wetzel: *"Confessions of a Cancer Conqueror"* is a tour de force of healing modalities in complimentary cancer care. Kirstin, a two-time cancer survivor, has walked the walk and offers her education, insights and experiences to help others find their own path to health. She explores the complex web of science, energy and thought as they relate to our individual well-being, and offers readers both a personal and professional perspective on the journey to health and healing.

Pat Wetzel, Founder and Member of *The Anti-Cancer Club* www.anticancerclub.com

Dana Ritchie: This is a GREAT book for people either trying to cope with or emerging from their cancer diagnosis about offering a clear self-help plan to make the required lifestyle changes to enable them a fighting chance at conquering this disease. What makes it endearing is that Kirstin infuses it with her own personal journey and holistic approach to finding a common thread that addresses the root causes that are unique to each of us. This book is based on evidence-based results combined with personal experience and offers huge value to all of us. Whether you have been diagnosed or are wishing to prevent becoming a statistic in the first place, this book is for you.

Dana Ritchie: bestselling author of *"The Ultimate Guide to Empower Yourself and Get What You Want in Life".*

FOREWORD

I wish this book had existed when I was diagnosed with my own breast cancer.

I was able to cure my own cancer naturally, but I spent hours and hours researching what I needed to do for myself. It was exhausting. You, dear reader, have the great blessing and good fortune of being able to use this book to create a plan to get you from just surviving to fully thriving. You will get all of the basics here in this book, plus have the opportunity to work with Kirstin to truly dial in your own individualized program to reverse your disease. What a gift!

I met Kirstin Nussgruber because of the circle of functional medicine health practitioners I love to spend my time with. She stood out because of the light that sparkles in her eyes and the passion that infuses her voice as she talks about how to prevent one of the most feared diseases in our culture – cancer.

Kirstin herself is an expert on this subject not only because she is thriving in spite of having gone through cancer two different times, but also because she has meticulously tested her research and interventions and come up with a dynamic program designed to benefit the millions of people touched by cancer in our country every year.

Cancer remains a leading cause of death in our world. Every year 12.7 million people are diagnosed with cancer and these rates are still on the rise. The sad truth is 30-40% of the 7.6 million people who actually die from cancer could have prevented it and 1/3 could be cured with early diagnosis and treatment.

The American Institute for Cancer Research and the World Cancer Research Fund say the very lifestyle factors outlined in this book can prevent as many as 340,000 American people from getting cancer each year. Kirstin provides you with specifics on food, exercise, and limiting the toxic load that is so prevalent in our environment today.

The truth is, the reasons people get cancer are the same reasons they get an autoimmune disease or any other chronic illness. There are four root causes to all of them: 1) genetics, 2) toxic exposure, 3) leaky gut, and 4) holding onto emotional wounds or past childhood trauma.

The ACEs Study (Adverse Childhood Experiences) that was conducted between 1995-1997 by Kaiser Permanente and the Centers for Disease Control illustrated the missing link between adult cancer and childhood trauma. Of the over 17,000 participants, over 2/3 reported at least one adverse childhood event, or they had an ACE Score of at least 1.

I have an ACE Score of 2. I have had both autoimmune disease and two forms of cancer. Past trauma is what I call the missing piece of the dis-ease puzzle. Stress and trauma are often given lip-service in the medical world, but little is done to offer concrete tools for reversing the impact of long-term stress and childhood trauma.

The great news is that an ACE Score of 1 or more does not mean disease is the automatic result. In fact, it's just the opposite. Neuroscience tells us the amazing healing power and plasticity of the brain is real and that it's possible to create new synaptic pathways no matter what your age.

The goal of overcoming trauma, healing leaky gut, detoxing, curing infections, and expressing your genetics differently boils down to one word: RESILIENCE.

By building resilience, you can reverse the ravages of stress, inflammation and yes...even cancer. Any program that teaches you to become more resilient in your body, heart, mind, and spirit is one worth doing. That is what Kirstin Nussgruber offers here in this valuable book.

Read it with hope, an open mind and a willingness to make the changes you will need to make in your life to turn this cancer train around. It can be done and I am so glad you have picked this book up.

Read on and may your life be filled with the joy and blessings of the gift that cancer ALWAYS brings...transformation.

Dr. Keesha Ewers

The bestselling author of "*Solving the Autoimmune Puzzle: The Woman's Guide to Reclaiming Emotional Freedom and Vibrant Health.*"

DEDICATIONS

LETTING GO

So this is it!
Here you are prepped for my own personal viewing.
Just you and me Mom.
One more time.
Despite the suffering edged on your face, you look incredibly peaceful,
even with a tightly shut mouth that appears forced.
I wasn't in time: I had to wait for the next flight. An ocean divided us,
yet it also gave me space over the years to gain perspective and mend
what needed to be healed.
I followed my instinct during the past sleepless nights; I sat and
meditated. I focused on you, on us, and felt the overwhelming urge to
give you permission to let go, to not wait for me.
What gets me is seeing you here, silent and waxy pale, and knowing
this is the final time we meet like this.
I clearly sense I am standing in front of the shell of your physical self,
of the embodiment you chose in this lifetime. While I am still in mine.
We are a lot more than an ocean apart now, and yet not.
You are released, free at last, and the tears that well up and start
pouring out are my relief from seeing this.
You are finally at peace, and we can connect on a different plane,

*because I became aware how, without the shackles of the ego, the
baggage of emotional wounds. I can finally tell you what you were
just not ready to hear from me, face-to-face.
How many times have we been at this threshold before, sometimes in
roles reversed, yet today is different.
No resentment. No hurt anymore. I understand. I get it this time.
Just pure love and forgiveness now. And ultimate peace.
I touch your cold body, and feel more connected to you
than ever before.*

(November 2010)

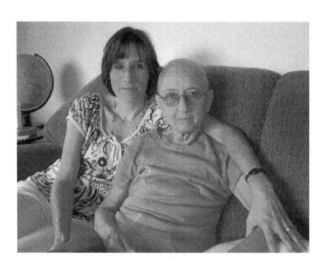

*Visiting my Mom after her second chemo, myself just
diagnosed a few days earlier*

To my Mom Christa, who loved me with all the love a mother can have for her child, and who made her decisions based on what she thought was the best thing to do at the time.

***

To my Aunt Helmtrud, who was the older sister I never had, and who succumbed to cancer way too soon relying solely on the crippling effects of conventional treatments, never giving up her smoking and staying trapped in a dysfunctional marriage.

***

To my Oma Anneliese, who at only 61 years old seemed like an ancient, disease-riddled woman to a nine year old girl who cried out of relief when she passed away because that meant an end to her intense suffering caused by decades of chronic medication that did not address any root causes of the autoimmune disease she was enslaved to since her early twenties.

Blessings and Inspirations

There are many beings I am truly blessed to have in my life, and without whose inspirational support I would not be the person I am today.

To my husband Claus, my rock to lean on, my sounding board to try out different tunes, my reality check, my ancient and wise soulmate, it still gives me the chills how deeply and solidly connected we are.

To my daughter Anita, whose bright and cheerful eyes and wise heart were the fuel that enabled me to break the chain that seemed to curse the female members of our family.

To my son Sven, whose quiet presence provided a depth of reassurance that enabled me to believe in the healing powers within me.

To my parents Christa and Dietger, who never gave up on answering my incessant "why?" questions, and who provided a nurturing home for me to grow up in.

To my extended family spread around the globe, who, although not ever-present in my life, still provide the glue that holds my world together and gives it meaning.

To the solid friendships that have stood by me during the rougher and vulnerable days when I needed their presence most of all.

To my teachers, colleagues and mentors who provided the backbone for catapulting me to become consciously aware of why I am here, and what I am capable of doing.

To the dogs (and cat) in my life over the last forty years, who first taught me what it means to be energetically connected and what unconditional love feels like.

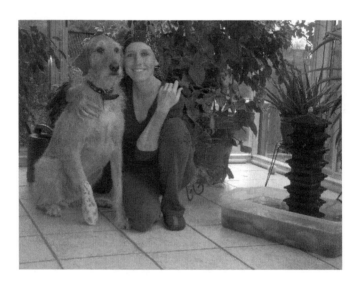

During Chemo #2 with one of my staunchest supporters, Duke, nursing a cut paw at the time

Why I wrote this book

"I learned that courage was not the absence of fear, but the triumph over it. The brave man is not he who does not feel afraid, but he who conquers that fear."
Nelson Rolihlahla Mandela

I am confronted with cancer on a daily basis.

Some may say "sure, because you professionally coach people that are in some way affected by cancer." While this is absolutely true, I am a cancer survivor, twice of breast cancer and also of skin cancer. And as survivors know, cancer is like a shadow that always follows us, if we allow it to be a shadow. And here is the key. We have a choice as to how we view this relationship we have with cancer.

It can be a dark shadow that we see as a disruptor of our happiness, dreams, ideals, and goals for a life we envisioned for ourselves. Or it can be something else entirely, something that may sound outrageous, if you are newly diagnosed, are battling through treatments or just emerging from the depths of the side effects and are wondering how the heck to continue with your life.

What if you could view cancer as a catalyst to a transformed You, as a gift or a blessing that led you down a path of discovery and opportunity you would never have imagined you would travel on, leading to a more enriched life than you have led until now, allowing you to find a new sense of Self Worth and helping you embrace a new purpose to your life?

If you are thinking "Never. How can this diagnosis ever be anything more than at worst a curse, and at best a total nuisance?" I can fully understand that. I have been through those exact sentiments on more than one occasion. Leaving that behind and moving onto a totally different mindset took guts, courage, tenacity, perseverance, a good dose of humor and a lot of personal navel gazing, coupled with plenty of emotional breakdowns.

I am the last one to tell you that the cancer journey is a straightforward path. It's a rough ride at times with numerous exasperating dead ends and turnarounds to explore another avenue. But, I will be the first to implore that every step you take to transform your relationship with your cancer is worth it.

Every cancer warrior needs support to walk this path, even if you are the one who chooses to face this demanding challenge in the comfort of your privacy.

I'm passionate about empowering you to explore your own path by offering you an insight in this book into what has helped my clients and me. My 5 Step Process to transform your relationship with cancer is meant to serve as a navigator along your path.

These 5 steps illustrate what resources we have at our disposal to embrace this journey we all start out with a battle, and which can end up uplifting us to unimaginable levels if we allow this to happen. Every one of us can conquer cancer, no matter at what stage we are at.

Let me offer you a glimpse into my journey so far.

I consider myself a "Third Culture" child, born and raised on different continents, exposed to the nuances of three different cultures, their languages and traditions. I learnt from a very young age how to adapt often and well to frequent change. Tearful farewells from close family and friends, and joyful reunions taught me to make the most of the present moment.

An only child, I was often the center of attention. While that had benefits, I was the main focus for a mother, who became increasingly frustrated and unfulfilled in her role of housewife. It caused many family conflicts and marital strife with me often sandwiched in between my parents.

It forced me to mature early. I became very sensitive to detecting other's needs and learnt to empathize to the point of sometimes being taken advantage of. It was isolating at times, and I turned to a self-survival strategy that would empower me to succeed in life. I became a bookworm and an academic achiever, acquiring knowledge was the tool that would help me do so, or so I thought, at the time.

Strong-willed, often impatient, and inquisitive to the point of annoying, I wanted to know the answers to everything, always counteracting an explanation with "Why" to dig deeper.

And I was always fascinated by food.

I grew up on canned veggies, Kraft spice blends and many packaged convenience foods. While my mother could cook tasty, I yearned for FRESH, and was quite a rebel when as a teenager I insisted on at least getting frozen veggies as an alternative to fresh, which my mother, going food shopping only once a month, would not entertain.

But, I also wanted to know how nutrition works for us. Although my earlier career had nothing to do with this, I educated myself along the way, turning my hobby into my new career at age 38 when I went back to school and attended the Zentrum für Naturheilkunde in Munich, Germany.

My family on my mother's side was riddled with chronic disease. Rheumatoid arthritis and cancer plagued the three women closest to me, my grandmother, my aunt and my mother. I grew up with the fear and emotional pain of seeing people I loved suffer. They all died way too young. I buried my Mom at age 68, so ravaged by disease that according to the funeral staff, she looked like she was in her 90's.

And then I myself was diagnosed with breast cancer at age 39. If there was one thing I knew immediately, it was this: I had no desire to go down the same path. I knew I needed to do a lot more than those three women close to me ever did to combat their disease. It was time to adapt again to change, resort to incessant questions, to go beyond the standard answers, and find the root causes that are not as obvious as they seem.

I owed this to myself, but also to my children. I remember how many people around me tried to soothe me by gently reminding me that cancer runs in my family, and that I was probably just a victim of circumstance, having done nothing wrong, so to speak.

Looking at the innocent and still very impressionable faces of my six-year-old daughter and ten-year-old son, I knew I owed them the fight for my life, but also for theirs. I needed to teach them the most important lesson a parent can convey, that getting to the root causes of any problem is the only way through it, and surrendering to voluntary ignorance or limited access to empowering knowledge is never an option.

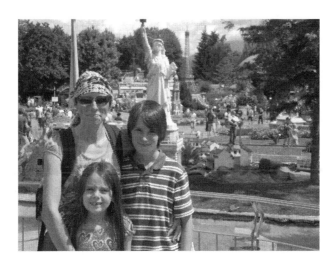

At Minimundus in Kärnten, Austria, using the in-between chemo phase to try and have a normal family life (2009)

This has been my passion ever since, to help myself thrive and share that with those who are intrigued and wish to do what it takes to thrive, themselves.

I realized that treating my body with conventional medicine alone was inadequate. Standard cancer treatments are only single-targeted therapies, concentrating exclusively on cancer cells in isolation from the rest of the body, ravaging the body's own healing power along the way. Many a cancer patient has become even more ill or died from the results of treatments such as chemotherapy and radiation taken too far.

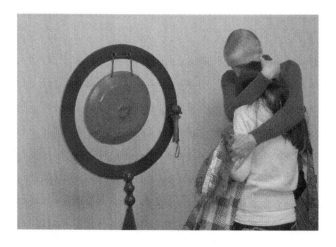

Hitting the gong after final radiation session #35 (2012)

I needed a multi-targeted approach, to focus on my whole being, and that meant addressing not just specific parts of the body, but acknowledging the dynamic inter-dependency of every single cell that makes up my body. This included focusing on the **mind** as well as the **soul**. These three dynamics, body, mind and soul, are interconnected and needed to be addressed with equal emphasis to determine the actual cause of my cancer, and facilitate true healing.

Most importantly, I recognized that **I alone was responsible for my health**, and could actively contribute to healing my body from cancer.

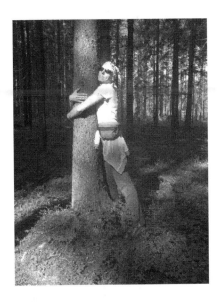

*Embracing the empowering energy of trees in the forest
near where we lived in Munich, Germany (2009)*

With the help of my family and friends, I endured the physical and emotional challenges of conventional treatments and their side effects, but I combined them with a **mindfulness approach** and **complementary forms of therapy**, some of which I still utilize today, and which I will discuss in this book.

Looking after my own health is a lifelong, fascinating and rewarding journey. Each of us carries within us an immense reservoir of inner strength and endurance.

I was determined to "**support my body**" with all the tools it required to heal itself, discovering the multitude of medicinal properties of whole, unprocessed foods, and targeted, high-quality supplementation, the ever present, but often dormant, conscious awareness that can be obtained with a calm and focused mind, the emotional healing that follows the release of unresolved inner conflicts and past trauma, acknowledging the role we can play in reducing our toxic burden in this modern society and utilizing the benefits of regular exercise.

I also realized that we are not just an intrinsic part of our environment; "**we are one with our environment**". Our body acts as a feedback mechanism. Our thoughts, attitudes and behavior have a direct impact on our health.

Most importantly, I am actively taking part in my healing process. I am deeply grateful for being given another chance, and am motivated to help educate and empower fellow cancer warriors, survivors like you, and anyone wishing to practice proactive prevention, to succeed in their own healing journey.

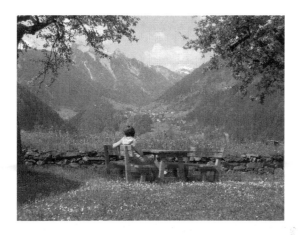

Looking out over the Zillertal, Austria, wig and all, on another in-between chemo trip that enabled me to gain new perspectives (2009)

"Changing is not just changing the things outside of us. First of all we need the right view that transcends all notions including of being and non-being, creator and creature, mind and spirit. That kind of insight is crucial for transformation and healing."
Thich Nhat Hanh

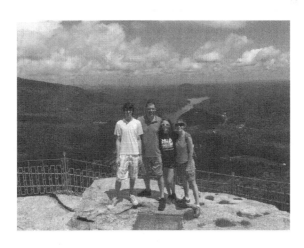

Climbing new peaks together at Lake Lure, NC (2016)

WHY YOU SHOULD READ THIS BOOK?

"If you don't like something, change it. If you can't change it, change your attitude."
Maya Angelou

When we are diagnosed with cancer, the shock of "becoming one of them," one of the brandished, the C-group or however we used to relate to people dealing with cancer before we were ourselves diagnosed, is stifling and almost overwhelming.

Cancer is so rampant in the westernized world these days that the silent fear that it might happen to us too is a little hazy cloud that we, if we are honest with ourselves, carry around with us wherever we go.

There are so many cancer stories these days that the facts and anecdotes almost become a blur. Stories of suffering through treatments, of miraculous recoveries using only alternative means, of recurrences after years of remission, and stories of true healing after conventional medicine had given a death timeline, abound and mingle with each other like guests at a cocktail party.

And now we have been invited to join this party called cancer.

I want you to know that what you may be feeling right now is absolutely normal. There is no right or wrong way; there is a sense of being overwhelmed, confused and there is this emotional wound that has been ripped open and is bleeding profusely and you may not know how to make it stop.

I want you to allow yourself some time to absorb and digest what is going on inside of you, and I hope this book will be a guide for you to win back your perspective, a bird's eye view that will enable you to make informed and empowering decisions so you can choose what will be the right path for you.

We are all on our own journey, and share this with no one else. Each of our cancers is unique to us, as cancer is so much more than just a pathological interpretation of the status of tissue gone malignant.

My hope is that this book helps clarify what your path needs to entail, and how you will select and fill your own unique healing toolbox from an array of options that holistically embrace your body, mind and soul. May you find your way within the 5 Step Process so you can succeed at transforming your relationship with cancer. For this is the key to unlocking the door to your very own healing path and personal self-discovery.

TABLE OF CONTENTS

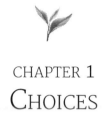

CHAPTER 1

CHOICES

"Today I choose life. Every morning when I wake up I can choose joy, happiness, negativity, pain... To feel the freedom that comes from being able to continue to make mistakes and choices – today I choose to feel life, not to deny my humanity but embrace it."
Kevyn Aucoin

If there is one thing I want to tell you right now as you stand at your own threshold of having to decide what to do, regardless of whether you have just been diagnosed, have completed treatments, or wish to prevent going down this road, it is this:

You have choices, and what worked best for me, and does for each of my clients, is to become familiar with the feeling of always having to choose. Even if you are unsure about whether it is the right thing to do.

While reading this you may be faced with treatment options and wondering which of the less than ideal choices is best for you. Do you follow the doctor's advice to the "T"? But, why is the doctor you consulted for a second or even third opinion recommending a different combination? How can you judge which one is right for you? After all, these are experts in their fields, who deal with this scenario daily.

I grew up with parents, who held doctors in such high esteem that they hardly questioned anything they said. It was a given that the Doc knows best. One was in awe of the White Coat and dared not appear disrespectful by "annoying" them with detailed questions.

I was an inquisitive child, and I am an inquisitive adult. I firmly believe that as a patient, you have the right to ask, politely of course, to understand the actual procedure that is recommended to you, the rationale behind it, what it wishes to achieve, what the success rate is and what you can expect to go through, short-term and long-term.

Next, upon receiving answers, how are they articulated and in what tone? Are you being treated with dignity and respect as an adult, on equal terms and at eye-level? Just because medical staff look official, dressed in coats with embroidered names, does not mean they have the right to assume your IQ, and capacity to memorize complex biological and medical terms, is below theirs.

When an electrician delivers an estimate for contract work to be done in your house, how do you feel toward him or her? Are you awe-struck by his or her detailed knowledge of a field of expertise that will forever remain beyond your mental grasp? Chances are, you aren't. You accept his or her expertise, but afford it the same credibility you wish to be shown, as the person, ultimately deciding whether to agree to the terms of the contract.

I am not suggesting you can negotiate a "better deal" with a doctor who is assisting you to make life-changing decisions, the extent of which you are not really qualified to fully understand. What I am suggesting is that you and the doctor are simply two people, equally respected and qualified in your own fields of expertise, engaging in a "contract" discussion which requires clarification on certain parts, and mutual respect as to the roles each of you will assume.

I vividly remember one doctor's response to a friend's question when she was confronted with having to choose a certain long-term hormone therapy regimen as an adjunct to her chemotherapy and radiation therapy, both of which she had already endured. She picked up on the "low libido" as a possible side effect, and wanted that clarified, as she explained that both her husband and herself were looking forward to being able to resume a normal sex life. The male doctor, much younger than my friend, who was in her forties, did not bother to look up from the paperwork he was scanning and simply said "well, what do you consider normal, once a day?"

If that had been me, I would have walked out. I would have fired him as my oncologist. We deserve better; we have a choice. We need to remember that we hire our doctors, and not the other way around.

Back to the never-ending slew of choices.

I want you to understand that you have the choice to decide how you deal with all these choices. The next step is crucial: accepting your choice and moving on, embracing how your life unfolds, taking stock to possibly re-evaluate and adjust your choices, add or drop some, but never chastising or judging yourself for making the choice you thought was the best for you at the time.

When I was diagnosed with my second, different, not recurrent breast cancer in three years, I went through a "guilt and blame" phase. You see, I had refused to receive radiation in addition to the chemotherapy and antibody (Herceptin) regimen I had already undergone, basing my decision at the time on my particular circumstances.

My first diagnosis at age 39 was a very early stage breast cancer, albeit HER2+ which only around 25% of breast cancers are. The Sentinel lymph nodes were clean. I was BRAC1 and BRAC2 negative and the surgeon had left conservative clean margins during the lumpectomy surgery, meaning he took out quite a bit more breast tissue than the actual tumor size, which was less than 1 cm, just to make sure.

Although I was ER (estrogen receptor) negative, but PR (progesterone receptor) positive, the oncologist suggested five years of hormone therapy with Tamoxifen, a drug which blocks estrogen receptors on breast cells. I also rejected this, considering it an over-kill and something which would drastically impact the quality of my life even more so than the surgery, chemo and Herceptin infusion had, a conclusion I came to after an extensive chat with a very empathetic female oncologist.

When the routine annual MRI three years later showed up a "slight enhancement", the mammogram and ultrasound did not confirm this. However, after the results of the thermography scan I insisted on having (outside the realm of conventional diagnostic tools, but I did it anyway because I was curious) indicated some inflammatory activity, I agreed to the MRI-guided biopsy.

The results confirmed malignant cells yet again. It threw me into an emotional tornado of betrayal, despair, but also tremendous guilt. What more did I need to do? Was it enough? Had I acted irresponsibly by refusing the additional recommended treatments three years previously? Had I caused this?

The abyss you fall into when emotionally doubting yourself should never be underestimated.

When describing this moment in my life, and going on to write about how I emerged from it and got myself grounded again, almost fails to capture just how emotionally volatile it is in this moment.

It is a moment that may last a few days, or for some, a few weeks. Whatever that time span, know that it is a normal phase of this journey we are thrust into as we discover the depths of ourselves, and just how strong we really are if we let ourselves hit rock bottom and are brave enough to look around.

When I regrouped and realized that this too is part of my journey and has some meaning even if it was still a mystery to me at the time, I also discovered this very important lesson: no matter what we decide to do to conquer our cancer, it is a choice we make, but it does not offer a guarantee. It offers us a chance at reclaiming our health. This can be different for each of us, and we need to first and foremost accept and embrace this life lesson.

You never go through the cancer experience alone, and besides family and friends, you may form bonds with fellow cancer warriors you meet who are going through the same or similar treatments at the same time.

I formed two such bonds during my first time, and it is to these individuals who I looked after I was diagnosed a second time.

We all had breast cancer and went through treatments, but all somewhat differently. Kate agreed to have all the conventional treatments that were offered, but also decided, like me, to simultaneously embrace a holistic approach.

She changed her eating habits, used energy healing sessions, cleared out her relationship closet and made some drastic changes, and focused on varied exercise. She is thriving today, travels the world and I frequently get a picture of her bundled up and smiling at the summit of a snow-peaked mountain, or dressed in pink as part of a team at a dragon boat race with a shiny gold medal around her neck.

Judith also followed her doctor's advice, but rejected any other supportive modality out of fear it may interfere with conventional treatments, unsupported by her traditional oncology team. She continued living her life as she had always done. She continued to bear the same emotional burdens and traumas (and there were quite a few) as before her diagnosis.

When I was last in touch with her, she was mentally and emotionally despondent and in daily physical pain, having had cancer recur three times, now fully metastasized. She suffered from the side effects of botched surgeries and was no closer to resolving her family trauma than when I first met her. Her initial oncologist, a renowned chief professor at a prestigious cancer center, had by then dismissed her case with the fine words "there is nothing more we can do for you".

I could go on, listing my clients' stories. The common thread that runs through all of them is this: we each make our choices, based on what we think to be the best at the time. Those of us who decide that we are in the driving seats of our cancer journeys generally fare much better and feel a lot more empowered and enabled to go beyond the visible surface and explore our unique root causes, ultimately facilitating true healing, whatever that may mean for us.

While Bernadette worked with me her cancer recurred and progressed rapidly. A successful attorney, she was generally very depressed and approached everything from a negative viewpoint. Slowly, we peeled off the layers and in between trying to cope with the physical symptoms of her disease progression, she had a moment where she realized what she had neglected to do all her life – address the root cause of why she felt so defeated about everything. She identified it as the psychologically abusive relationship she had as a single mother with her now adult son.

She candidly remarked she wished she had met me earlier on her journey, realizing it was now too late to hope for a physical recovery miracle, but was making peace with what this meant for her despite having no hope from receiving any compassion from her son, even in her last week at hospice when we last communicated with each other.

Choosing to accept, confront, embrace and transform your relationship with cancer is the one thing that you do have ultimate power over, regardless of which other choices you may find yourselves confronted with. As you continue reading this book, you will find me listing some options you can use to turn this challenging diagnosis around into a life-enhancing experience, if you are willing to look at it this way.

What follows is not a reference-style list of all the choices you have at your disposal to help you achieve this mindset. Rather, I want you to gain the perspective of five distinct areas where you can find some answers that will help you find your own path to reclaiming your life.

I need to make one important point though. When it comes to the five-step process to transform your relationship with cancer, it is not about choosing which step applies to you. If you really want to get to the root cause, you need to address all five in an ongoing way.

Of course, there will be choices within each area, and more than I will list here. I will guide you to a baseline understanding on how to get started right after you have finished reading this book.

Welcome to the transformative journey that will redefine your life!

CHAPTER 2

WHY CANCER CAN GAIN A FOOTHOLD IN THE FIRST PLACE

"For me the greatest beauty always lies in the greatest clarity."
Gotthold Ephraim Lessing

When I was first diagnosed with breast cancer, the question that seemed to flash before me incessantly like a bright neon light was this: "Did my genetic flaws really cause my cancer?"

There is a history of breast cancer in my immediate family. It seems obvious that that places me in a higher risk category, and when the moment comes, one can easily put it down to "it's my turn now."

Intuitively, I wanted to dig deeper, and find answers to whether or not someone with a genetic history of cancer has no other resources than to simply hope to be the lucky one, who escapes the family curse. This would lead me to discover perhaps whether or not there is something someone like me could have done, or can still do, to redirect what appears to be an inevitable genetic pathway.

What also intrigued me, was to find out whether there is a common root cause underlying what triggers, drives and fuels cancer, irrespective of which organ the original tumor is found in, and whether or not there is a genetic history.

I also found myself seriously asking for the first time why we as a society are still so challenged when it comes to finding "the cure".

From a medical point of view, to date, there is still no guaranteed cure for cancer. The magic bullet in conventional treatments that the medical establishment has been striving for for decades, does not yet seem to exist.

When I was one year old, in 1971, President Nixon infamously declared war on cancer by signing the National Cancer Act as cancer was the second leading cause of death in the US at that time, being surpassed only by deaths from heart disease. Since then hundreds of billions of dollars have been spent on cancer research and treatments worldwide. Despite this, the statistics have not shifted much.

According to a 2015 report by the US National Center for Health Statistics based on 2014 data, cancer still accounted for 591,699 deaths, only surpassed by heart disease at 614,348. Almost fifty years later, the CDC (Center for Disease Control & Prevention) in the US appealed for a proactive approach to fight this disease and find solutions that apparently seem to be imminent.

Why are we still struggling with this, notwithstanding the fact that medical treatment options have improved drastically over these past five decades?

The conventional way of approaching cancer is to target the tumor or cancer cells only, not the whole body, or the real underlying cause. Inroads are, however, being made in the fairly new cancer treatment domain of immunotherapy, where the focus is on supporting the body's immune system to do what it essentially is supposed to do on its own. However, clinical trials are still in progress, and years away from allowing these less invasive treatments to be offered as a standard approach to replace the often debilitating current treatments such as chemotherapy and radiation therapy that systematically weaken the entire body.

Cancer does not exist in isolation; it is influenced by its surrounding environment and can actively communicate between cells. Scientists and researchers have known this for over a century.

In most cases, cancer is a disease from within your body. It is a process that although seems confined to a particular area, affects your entire body. We can try and intervene at the point where it seems visible, such as a tumor site, but that is not addressing the actual cause, simply treating the symptom.

There is one underlying commonality for all cancers, no matter what body part it shows up in, your cells start misbehaving, a bit like unruly rebellious teenagers, who think only of their immediate gratification and fail to comprehend the consequences of their actions on their surroundings.

Normal cells have a specific purpose; they divide if they have to, perform their specific function and die off when they have finished their task or duty for the entire good, a process referred to as apoptosis.

Cancer cells do not adhere to rules for the common good. They trick the body into actually supporting their growth and progression.

A normal body has a solid self-defense and protection mechanism. When there is inflammation in a particular area in the body, your immune system gets activated and sends in its agents to repair or replace any damage. Have you ever wondered why, when you cut yourself, the area becomes swollen, red and sore? This is your body's response to providing healing support, sending in the troops via different types of white blood cells to fight potential pathogens and offer cell repair to close a wound. Simply put, this is direct evidence of simple cellular communication to get the job done.

Cancer cells can disrupt this communication. They can simulate the natural healing process and use it to their advantage, for example to attract resources such as its own blood vessel supply, a process referred to as angiogenesis. The simple instruction given is "Help me grow!"

Cancer cells can influence their surrounding environment by making it more penetrable and allowing a tumor to spread, a process called tumor progression. The simple instruction given is "Help me spread!"

Cancer cells can prevent natural cell death, a process referred to as apoptosis, thereby giving the instruction "Help me become invincible!"

And cancer cells can neutralize your immune system through overstimulation, exhausting it in the process so that it is unable to detect and fight off cancer growth.

What flips the switch?

A common, generalized answer sounds something like this: you are in a way predestined through any of the following factors in your life, such as bad genes, lifestyle choices, exposure to environmental factors, and outside pathogens and viruses.

What puzzled me about this explanation is why everyone exposed to identical factors within these above categories, does not get cancer.

There must be something else within each of us that can promote or deter cancer development and progression even if exposed to the same or very similar environmental conditions.

I'd like to take a little scientific detour to help you understand what resources we indeed have at our disposal to become an active participant in influencing our internal environment. I have highlighted only two existing theories, not because I think they are the all-inclusive answer, but they make a lot of sense to me, and underline the power we have to influence possible underlying common causes of cancer.

Theory of gene expression

Every cell in your body has all the genetic information required to create you. This is referred to as your genome. It is inherited and considered fixed, but this does not mean your destiny is fixed!

Not all of these genes are being expressed, or activated, at any given moment. Scientists have found that each gene has certain chemical tags, called epigenomes, which tell a gene what to do, and when to do it. This essentially is gene expression, and can be influenced by your choices.

Fascinating research has been done in the field of nutritional epigenetics which looks at what nutritional factors determine how much or whether genes are expressed. It has been discovered that we have both tumor-suppressing as well as cancer-promoting genes. (Bishop, KS, Ferguson, LR, 2015).

Something turns these genes either on or off, and that something that turns cancer-promoting genes on has been discovered and labeled as cancer's master switch, Nuclear Factor-kappa Beta (NFkβ), a signaling molecule that, if activated, causes inflammation and inhibits cancer cell death or apoptosis. (Aggarwal BB, 2002,2004).

NFkβ can activate a few hundred genes that promote either tumor survival through angiogenesis, proliferation and invasion. NFkβ can be activated by cellular inflammation, toxicity (also from chemotherapy and radiation), other carcinogens and prolonged exposure to stress.

It makes sense to want to control NFkβ, make it inactive or at least dormant. Incidentally, the pharmaceutical industry has been researching the possibility of inhibiting the expression of NFkβ. (Lee CH et al. 2007).

However, according to the research, stocking your spice cabinet with certain anti-inflammatory and anti-oxidant rich spices, such as turmeric, cinnamon, ginger, cloves, nutmeg, cardamom and black pepper can go a long way towards actively modulating the expression of NFkβ. (Ichikawa H et al. 2008).

In particular, the active compound curcumin in turmeric has been studied extensively, and has been shown actually to inhibit NFkβ. Certain countries, such as India, have been shown to have lower overall cancer rates, a fact that is contributed, in part, to their higher and much more varied spice intake.

You can also influence the process by which a gene can express itself. The chromosomes within a gene need to undergo a change when a cell divides (become unwrapped and unzipped), and this change can be influenced by a myriad of compounds within some specific food groups. More on this later in the book.

So, the gene expression theory can explain why everyone with a genetic mutation does not necessarily end up getting cancer.

But is there a common cause, something that all cancers seem to have in common?

This may have been answered almost one hundred years ago.

Theory of cancer as a mitochondrial disease

Each cell in our body can produce energy for our body as a whole to survive. Cells do this through a mechanism that uses oxygen and a fuel in the form of glucose or fat.

The process by which the oxygen gets to each cell, and then is made available to the cell, and turned into energy, can be damaged, and seems to be an underlying commonality in all cancers.

In 1931 the Nobel Prize was awarded to German researcher Dr. Otto Warburg, who stated over 80 years ago, that cancer cells use energy differently than healthy cells, namely via the sugar fermentation process. This allows them to produce energy without having oxygen present, but requires a lot more glucose than a normal cell. It is a lot less efficient, but ensures their survival, nevertheless.

You may be familiar with this theory, as it is used in medical diagnostic tests. Most cancer patients are required to undergo a PET scan once initially diagnosed, to rule out any possible metastasized cancer tumors in different locations in the body. Before the scan, you are injected with radioactively labeled glucose that will be quickly absorbed by cancer cells. The point of a PET scan is to find areas where glucose is taken up at a much faster rate than elsewhere, indicating the presence of an active tumor.

Dr. Thomas Seyfried, a leading cancer researcher at Yale University & Boston College, expanded in the last few years upon Dr. Warburg's almost century-old theory.

Simply put, all cells use glucose (sugar) as fuel and oxygen to produce energy in a very specific place inside the body, the mitochondria, which are tiny cell organelles inside each cell.

These mitochondria can become damaged through inherited mutations, environmental factors and toxins, and it is the extent of this damage that, if left unchecked, can escalate and over time lead to cellular dysfunction and tumor development.

Dr. Heinrich Kremer, MD, a German cell symbiosis researcher and author of *"The Silent Revolution in Cancer and Aids Medicine,"* explains: "mitochondria produce energy via two pathways: with the help of oxygen and with the help of glucose, regulated via an automatic switch mechanism."

A normal cell does two things with this energy: it performs its specific function, and it divides itself when it needs to. The energy generated with the help of oxygen allows the cell to perform its specific function. The instruction given is Work! The energy generated with the help of glucose is used only during normal cell division. The instruction given is Divide!

Damaged mitochondria do not switch back and forth between these two modes of energy production. They get stuck in the glucose – energy mode, essentially stuck in the divide mode, reproducing uncontrollably.

Dr. Johannes Coy, a German chemist, elaborates on this glucose theory by confirming that normal, healthy cells burn glucose during energy production, whereas cancer cells ferment glucose with the help of an enzyme, TKTL-1 enzyme (Transketolase-like 1 enzyme).

He found this enzyme is present in various types of cancer. It allows cancer cells to ferment glucose even in the presence of oxygen. The fermentation process produces lactic acid that changes the surrounding environment of the cells, making it dependent on glucose for fuel, and allowing cancer to invade neighboring territory.

According to these theories, cancer is the process where a normal cell is damaged and produces energy purely through sugar fermentation. This is not an efficient way of producing energy, so the cell essentially does not have enough energy available to perform its usual tasks and only divides without inhibition.

This can further lead to genetic changes, leaving a cell that is no longer a highly specialized unit, but has to cut back and resort to a more primitive level of existence. Pure survival, divide and grow. Period. No more communication between other cells. This, according to this line of thought, is cancer.

Now, where does that leave you? If you are like me, I am pretty sure you want to switch off the process of cell damage called cancer.

Let's understand that we have choices and that a combined effort of many of them can actively contribute to creating an environment that is unwelcoming to cancer growth.

CHAPTER 3

STEP 1
EAT SMART, NOT JUST RIGHT

"Your diet is a bank account. Good food choices
are good investments."
Bethenny Frankel

I grew up on canned veggies and only really began experimenting with fresh food once I had my own kitchen. One of the first
things I bought was a salad spinner. Being on a limited budget, it
was a cheap plastic item that distorted when spinning, but nevertheless lasted nearly ten years.

When I was diagnosed years later I thought we, as a family were
pretty healthy eaters. We had a balanced diet; we were all slim
and weight was never an issue. However, when I began studying
functional nutrition, I discovered what it truly takes to nourish
our body fully.

It is not just about what we eat, but also about what conditions could be simmering underneath the surface, even with a
"healthy diet". It is also about what support our body needs to

convert what we offer it into fuel it can use, without creating a host of byproducts that can harm our delicate biochemistry.

Our bodies are magnificent wonders: they are robust enough to withstand harsh physical pressure and stress, able to bounce back and, with help, reconnect torn muscles, ligaments, vessels and sometimes even nerves. Nowadays, we can exchange body parts and the body will generally not reject what is essentially a foreign object. They are also so fine-tuned to regulate microscopic nerve signaling to ensure an intricate communication exchange that would rival the interconnected highway systems of large cities around the globe.

Nourishing our bodies is a way of honoring them and paying tribute to the myriad of automatic, and invisible functions we take for granted to keep us alive. It is our duty to ensure that what we eat is pure, nutrient rich and in a format that our own body can easily identify and use.

It is also our duty to ensure that our body can use this fuel in the correct way. Supporting our entire digestive system, and monitoring whether our cells are actually absorbing all the macro as well as micronutrients, while ensuring we are not deficient in any, is equally as important as putting the right food on our plate. And once again, this can be different for you and me.

Reconnecting with Real Food

Healthy nutrition is a very important subject, but it can be very confusing and overwhelming as there are so many theories and diet-styles available to choose from.

In this book I seek to provide a solid understanding of the very basics of an anti-cancer way of eating, regardless of which particular dietary direction you choose to follow. I could write an entire encyclopedia on real nutrition, however that is not the scope of this book. I want you to walk away with some tips you can implement right away, and successfully turn into daily habits.

As cancer warriors, we need to grasp how our food choices influence cancer growth overall, and to realize that once we do this, we can still choose to eat in a particular way, depending on our bio-individuality.

There is no one right way to eat for everybody as we have to take our own unique physiology and sensitivities into account. However, there is a right way to make cancer-fighting choices that form the basis for the many different dietary directions we can choose to adopt.

I am not about to tell you that you have to follow a certain single diet, but there is a certain way of mindful and educated eating that I support, because it makes absolute sense, and is supported by current scientific research. My goal is to introduce you to choices when you decide what to put on your cancer-fighting plate. And choices you have, lots of them!

Science knows that cancer cells have a much higher concentration of insulin receptors on their membranes, as they require copious amounts of glucose to accommodate for their inefficient way of producing cellular energy. Insulin is the hormone produced by the pancreas, which acts as a key for glucose, allowing it to fit the lock to the door called cell membrane and granting access into the cell.

We also know that cancer thrives in an inflammatory environment as this weakens the natural cell defense mechanisms and creates an environment in which cancer cell growth can more easily go undetected.

And we also know that there are ways to influence the switching on or off of cancer-promoting or cancer-suppressing genes. Having these genetic defects does not mean they will inevitably trigger cancer growth. Something still needs to activate them. Nutrition is one of the areas where we can influence this.

Is my sugar intake fueling my cancer?

This is a standard question that every single client asks; it is also a question I had when I was diagnosed, even though I was not a sugar monster, or so I thought. Ditching sugar was something I found comfort in, as unbelievable as this may sound, at the time, I felt it gave me something to do to actively tackle my cancer cells.

But, let's not jump to conclusions and make rash decisions that do not address the whole picture.

Sugar is a little more complex than the white fluffy or liquid corn-derived stuff we have come to buy and consume in increasing quantities in the western world.

Sugar is not just a finished end-product. In the molecular form of glucose it is also a by-product of a breakdown of the foods we eat, mainly carbohydrates, or "carbs" as we generally refer to them, from products made of wheat flour (such as bread, cakes, pastries and pasta) as well as fresh foods such as starchy root vegetables.

Our body needs glucose for energy production, and certain

organs, in particular our brain, depends on this form, or so we generally think. Our body has developed a mechanism to stock its pantry when there is an excess to accommodate for glucose shortages in times of need.

Glucose can be converted to glycogen, which is stored mainly in the liver and to a lesser extent also in the skeletal muscles. If these storage chambers are filled to capacity, any excess glucose is stored as fat, and this storage capacity does not offer natural limitations, leading to obesity if left unchecked.

Conversely, if all glycogen and glucose is depleted, the body will set a different mechanism in action, reserved exclusively for survival, by extracting glucose from non-carbohydrate sources such as proteins, in a process called gluconeogenesis.

This is not a very efficient process; it can result in the breaking down of muscle fibers and resultant muscle wasting, evidence of this is seen in emaciated victims of starvation. Low-carbo-hydrate diets or periods of intense exercise can also lead to the body obtaining the glucose it needs from gluconeogenesis.

Another survival mechanism can also kick in in times of low carb exposure, called ketosis - the underlying mechanism of a ketogenic diet. This is when the body switches its energy supply to what is called a state of ketosis, by obtaining most of its fuel from fat, thereby releasing and using so-called ketones. Ketones are made in the liver from fat if there is a very low carb and insulin supply, as well as a low protein supply. Ketones will replace glucose as fuel for your body, including your brain. So, essentially, your brain can function without glucose if you keep your body in a consistent state of ketosis.

A quick note on the ketogenic diet as this form of eating falls into the category of an anti-cancer diet and you may encounter many who swear by it, and have seen great metabolic results from it, including weight loss and healthy weight management.

Each of us needs to find what works best for our bodies. I am not a friend of exclusively following any specific diet. We need to practice caution as every diet has very strict rules, the ketogenic diet in particular, and may need to be monitored by a professional and requires certain lab tests. It may not be the right way of eating for your physiology, and many clients have come to me after embarking on a variety of strict diets, wondering why they are not feeling well.

Does it make sense then, to say the easiest way to starve cancer cells is to cut out all sugar? I believe that this is too simplistic a view, and if that were the case, cancer would have been eradicated by now. Cutting out all dietary sugar alone is not just the issue. Rather, if the body cannot manage normal blood sugar levels, it can trigger a cascade of inflammatory responses that can create an environment we may not necessarily become aware of until it is in an advanced state. This environment can potentially fuel cancer growth.

The Sugar issue becomes the CARB issue

To understand how we can unknowingly create and nurture this cancer-fueling environment, let's revisit how our body utilizes carbohydrates, Carbs, from sources such as bread, pasta, rice, flour products, crackers, pastries, cakes, and starchy root vegetables, are the energy suppliers for the body. When you consume carbs, they are digested and converted to glucose in the blood that then needs to be transported into each cell. This is done via the hormone insulin.

If glucose levels in the blood are too high, more insulin is secreted by the pancreas. But, if due to poor dietary choices, there is a constant spike in blood sugar levels, this insulin-glucose regulating system can, over time malfunction, leading to constantly elevated glucose and insulin levels.

This stresses the body and can create an inflammatory reaction referred to as insulin resistance, which can provide an environment in the body that favors tumor growth and progression. It is a leading underlying cause of rampant Diabetes II. Unlike Diabetes I where the body simply cannot produce any insulin, here the body has ample supply, but it has become ineffective.

Besides leading to a high blood sugar level, having a constant oversupply of insulin in your blood is bad news for another reason. Insulin itself acts as a growth factor through the hormone IGF-1 (Insulin-like growth factor). A study in 2008 to test the growth-promoting actions of insulin showed that babies with type 1 diabetes and the resulting hypoinsulinemia (insufficient insulin) had shorter bone growth than obese children with hyperinsulinemia (chronic elevated insulin levels), who were taller, with longer bone growth.

Science knows that high levels of IGF-1 can lead to growth and cell differentiation, so as a cancer-prevention strategy, ensuring that we do not have excess insulin floating around, is a smart move!

What can cause insulin resistance?

We need to understand that insulin resistance is a lifestyle-induced condition, and can thus be reversed. Besides consuming too many simple carbs and refined sugar products, other factors can contribute to insulin resistance too, such as deficiencies in those nutrients that regulate blood sugar levels which include Vitamin D, magnesium, zinc, chromium, conjugated linoleic acid and biotin.

Stress, a lack of sleep, as well as lack of physical exercise and poor digestion can also contribute. Muscle wasting is a side effect of cancer treatments such as chemotherapy and radiation. Muscle loss can lead to imbalanced blood sugar levels as muscles themselves take up excess glucose and store it in the form of glycogen.

Signs of insulin resistance

If you show any two or more of these signs, you need to address your blood sugar level (drweil.com/metabolic syndrome, 2013). Please note these are lab reference ranges, and you need to always take your individual circumstances into account.

➤ Waist circumference: at least 35 inches for women and at least 40 inches for men

➤ Fasting blood glucose at least 100 mg/dL

➤ Serum triglycerides at least 150 mg/dL

➤ Blood pressure at least 135/85mmHg

➤ HDL ("good") cholesterol lower than 40 mg/dL for men or 50 mg/dL for women

---

How can you balance blood sugar nutritionally?

Here's a simple rule: you can eat certain foods and avoid others!

Certain foods get converted to sugar at a much faster rate than others. This raises your blood sugar level quickly. You can test this when you are really hungry and grab whatever comes to hand first, which is usually a bar, a bagel, a cookie, a muffin. You feel better, your system is flooded with glucose, yay, energy real fast!

But, then a short while later you feel tired and irritable again, the typical blood sugar dip. A quick rush of energy, but nothing to sustain it over a longer period.

Now the more fiber you consume, the slower the digestion process, the slower the release of glucose, the slower the rise of your blood sugar in a way your body can handle it and process it. A steady supply of energy, no ups and downs, no fatigue, no feeling sluggish.

This is what you want to achieve. Eating food that supplies a steady blood sugar level, and a fool-proof method is to eat foods high in fiber. This applies to food in its most natural state as well as to processed food.

Let me give you a quick list of the top "sugar" offenders, that if regularly consumed — by that I mean a few times each day — contribute to constantly keeping your blood sugar levels spiked.

You want to either limit or avoid

1. Refined sugar products (check labels for all forms, including white, brown, corn syrup, High Fructose Corn Syrup, and the –oses such as sucralose, dextrose, maltodextrose, fructose).

2. Refined carb products made from white flour such as cereals, crackers, pasta, pastries, bread, cake.

3. Alcohol (approximately 2 drinks/week for women and 4 drinks/week for men is acceptable – treat it as a treat rather than a routine staple).

4. Limit fruits to max 2–3 servings/day.

5. Dried fruits, over–ripe bananas with brown spots on them.

6. All sweetened drinks including sodas, fruit juices, iced teas and flavored waters.

A note on fruit. Some fruits are high in sugars, mainly fructose, such as melons, bananas, pineapple, mangoes. You should not be avoiding these fruit as they are rich in vital nutrients and enzymes plus have a healthy dose of fiber to slow down the blood sugar rush.

If you happen to be sensitive to fructose, which you can find out via a functional test, then it is prudent to limit the intake of these to no more than 2/3 times per week. Fructose is metabolized differently in the body to glucose, and can lead to high triglyceride levels (unhealthy fat ratio). Better choices for a daily intake of fruits include green apples and pears, certain stone fruits such as apricots, peaches, plums, pomegranates, and berries such as blueberries, raspberries, strawberries, blackberries. Fruit overall, provides a key element in the cancer-fighting "Eat Rainbow" strategy, more on that later.

Sugar improves the shelf life and flavor and is, therefore, added to most of the packaged foods we find on supermarket shelves. Don't be fooled by low-fat or any "light" products, as they only have any flavor because of the added sugars, giving back flavor that the lack of fat has taken out. Going "fat-free" to eat healthily is one of the largest misconceptions the food industry bestowed upon us during the 80's and 90's. It led to a rise, not a decline, in obesity, diabetes II, cardiovascular disease, strokes and heart attacks.

Even though you may wish to avoid all processed foods altogether, let's be honest, we have to consume some processed foods, so let's learn how we can be smart about which ones we choose.

Check the Nutrition Facts labels!

When you pick up a packed food item, what is the first thing you do? You tend to immediately look at the sugar content, correct? I do. My first "go-to." How much sugar, and in what form. Let's explore that a little, as there is more to this than "just" the sugar content, if you want to become a savvy label reader.

How much sugar is acceptable? A simple rule is to be wary of any amount of 6-10g of sugar or more. And here's the catch - in the amount you want to eat - not in the labeled serving size! There is a big difference as some serving sizes are so small you would eat

2 or 3 times that amount if eating that entire product.

Is the sugar content easy to identify? Anything that includes the word "sugar" is pretty easy to spot, and so is honey instantly recognizable, as well as the "syrups" including maple syrup, malt syrup, brown rice syrup, corn syrup, and high-fructose corn syrup.

There are so-called "hidden" sugars - fructose, glucose, lactose, maltose, dextrose, maltodextrin, barley malt, molasses, evaporated cane juice, fruit juice, and fruit juice concentrate.

A quick note on the infamous high fructose corn syrup (HFCS). This sugar substitute is synthetically derived, much sweeter and cheaper to produce than sugar; it is banned in the European Union. The main issue is its high fructose content. I mentioned earlier, that fructose has a different structure to other sugar molecules, and is metabolized differently in the body, being mainly converted to fat. It raises insulin levels faster as well as uric acid levels, which affects blood pressure and kidney function. By consistently consuming HFCS – and this is easily done with US processed foods, in particular sodas, our uric acid levels could constantly be elevated, a factor which is seen by the functional medicine world as a more powerful risk factor in determining heart disease than cholesterol.

What about artificial sweeteners? They are synthetic and can have toxic effects on the body. A big NO. Take the ingredient Aspartame. When it is broken down in the body one of the by-products is formaldehyde. This can accumulate in our cells and cause damage to the DNA, which can potentially lead to cells mutating.

Aspartame is also an excitotoxin; it can cross the blood-brain barrier and damage the brain and nervous system. Some artificial sweeteners have been shown to cause other disruptive effects, one of which being able to reduce the amount of good bacteria in the gut.

The go-to sweetener is Stevia, a herbal extract which is calorie-free and does not cause any blood sugar or insulin rise. It comes in powder or liquid form, which I personally prefer, and it is 100 times sweeter than sugar. One drop used to be enough to sweeten my bowl of oatmeal, when I was still weening myself off the habit of having to sweeten it lightly. I do not use it in my green or herbal tea, or occasional treat coffee, as I have systematically weaned myself off having to sweeten most of my foods. It took me a while. You need to allow your taste buds to adjust slowly if you want to sustain long term success. Now, I love the more bitter taste and cannot take a sweetened beverage.

Let's get back to our nutrition labels and on becoming savvy label readers.

Two other crucial ingredients on that food label demand our attention, the amount of total carbohydrates and fiber. These provide a far more accurate assessment of how quickly that sugar content will cause your blood sugar level to rise, whether or not this will stress – or not – your insulin production and over time, if consumed on a regular basis, add to cellular inflammation, insulin resistance and an environment which favors cancer cell growth.

Here is another simple rule you can apply to enable you to make the decision of whether to grab and go or rather leave on the shelf. Compare the total carbohydrates number with the fiber number, and apply the 10:1 rule: for every 10g of total carbs listed, there should be at least 1g of dietary fiber to balance your blood sugar.

I want to illustrate the 10:1 rule with a few examples (brand names are withheld):

Energy Bar, Choc Chip flavor, serving size 1 bar

> ➤ Total carbs: 44g (of which 23g are sugars)
> ➤ Fiber: 4g

Apply 10:1 rule: 44:4
Verdict: just makes it into the "acceptable" range, but the sugar content is way too high.

Granola Bar, serving size 1/3 cup

> ➤ Total carbs: 20g (of which 6g are sugars)
> ➤ Fiber: 2g

Apply 10:1 rule: 20:2
Verdict: just makes it into the "acceptable" range, and the sugar content is below the 10g limit.

Store-bought orange juice, serving size: 8 fl oz or 240 ml (about 1 glass)

> ➤ Total carbs: 26g (of which 23g are sugars)
> ➤ Fiber: none!

Apply 10:1 rule: can't!
Verdict: this is a sugar bomb! Severely dilute it, limit or avoid altogether and replace with a real orange!

The revised Nutrition Facts Label, which was introduced by the FDA (Food and Drug Administration) in 2014 to provide a more accurate ingredient information on packaged foods, has some great updates, the most important ones being

- the serving size is more realistic now, it is larger and thus will show a higher calorie value

- trans fats have to be shown – aim for 0!

- total fat content has to be noted – aim for 5% or less, no more

- 10:1 Rule (Total carbs to fiber, see the previous chapter)

- keep an eye out for sodium content. Keep within a 5% range, no more. The total daily amount for an adult should be limited to around 2.3 g (2,300 mg). 1 teaspoon of table salt is a little over that! (US Dept of Health & Human Services' Office of Disease Prevention & Health Promotion)

Categorizing real food – understanding the Glycemic Index and Glycemic Load

Let's turn our attention to real, whole foods. How do we know which ones get converted faster into glucose, thereby raising our blood sugar levels, and which don't?

There is a system that helps you figure out how whole foods affect your blood sugar levels, which uses 2 measuring and categorization tools – the Glycemic Index and Glycemic Load.

The Glycemic Index (GI) indicates the quality of the carbs you eat. It rates how quickly your blood sugar level rises when eating certain single foods. The standard rating against which each food is measured is a teaspoon of table sugar, which equals 100. Then a score of between 0 and 100 is applied to each food.

A high GI score is above 80. Refined sugar, refined carbs & white flour products fall into this category. A moderate GI score is between 60-80. Whole grain products and whole grains such as rice, quinoa, barley, buckwheat, millet, amaranth can be found here. A low GI score is under 60. Most vegetables, protein, nuts, seeds, legumes can be found here.

A combination of foods also affects the GI. For example, eating a moderate or high GI food together with a low GI food

slows down glucose release, thus not spiking the blood sugar level too quickly.

Food preparation too can affect the GI. For example, according to www.nutritiondata.self.com, a large baked potato, with skin ranks around a GI of 29, boiled in skin the GI drops to 7, 1 cup mashed with whole milk added it becomes a GI of 16.

The Glycemic Load (GL) indicates the quantity of the carbohydrates you eat. It takes into consideration how many carbs you eat, whether you eat them alone or with food that slows down digestion such as fiber, protein and healthy fats. A good rule to follow is never eat carbs alone! Always make sure you include an additional vegetable or food high in fiber, a protein source and a healthy fat. For example, dipping starchy root vegetables such as carrots, kohlrabi, turnips or jicama root in a hummus dip gives you a perfectly balanced GL.

A word of caution though, the GI and GL system is a v̇
way of balancing your food intake to help you figure ouᴛ
are managing your blood sugar levels effectively to avoid feᴇ
into an underlying inflammatory condition referred to as insulin
resistance. Best use it as a guideline only, not as a new dogma to
measure out every single food item you consume. This can very
easily overwhelm and rob you of the joy of eating.

Once you familiarize yourself with a basic category of low, moderate and high glycemic foods, it will become second nature to
you and you will soon find yourself adept at selecting foods and
combining balanced meals on your own.

*Would a basic **BALANCE YOUR BLOOD SUGAR** Cheat
Sheet listing the GI of some common foods be helpful?
I have one for you to download right now!
Click here if you are reading a digital book version*

*http://www.kirstinscancercare.com/balance-blood-sugar-
cheat-sheet/*

or find it at
http://www.kirstinscancercare.com/awesomebookbonuses/

Why FATS are an essential component of an anti-cancer way of eating

Mention the word "fats" today and many people cringe and want
to run in the opposite direction. Fats received such a bad rap in
the late 80's and into the 90's, when all and sundry went fat-
free, processed food lost a lot of its flavor and became rampant

35

with added sugars to compensate for this. Coincidentally, the use of anti-depressants almost trebled between 1988 and 2000. (Source: CDC National Center for Health Statistics Press Office).

Our bodies need fat; it fuels our nervous system and our brain is dependent upon it. Certain fat-soluble vitamins are dependent upon it for proper absorption, in particular, Vitamin D as a deficiency is also linked to depression.

However, we need to become very aware of the type of fats we eat, as well as the ratio of the fats we eat. Put very simply, the fats we eat end up as part of our cell membranes. There they affect the consistency of the actual cell membrane which allows nutrient and waste exchange – food in, waste out, pretty similar to us humans.

Fats are also converted into chemical messengers (eicosanoids), which are either pro-inflammatory, and thus harmful, or anti-inflammatory and thus beneficial.

Omega 6 fats can act as precursors for potent pro-inflammatory molecules such as prostaglandin E2 and leukotriene B4. These have been shown to stimulate tumor growth (through angiogenesis), promote proliferation of tumors and suppress immune function.

They can be found in commercially raised meat, poultry, dairy, eggs as well as nuts such as walnuts, almonds, pecans, undyed pistachios, brazils, and in particular, in sunflower seeds and pumpkin seeds. An important side note is that vegetable-sourced Omega 6 fats can be converted to beneficial anti-inflammatory prostaglandin E1.

Omega 3 fatty acids are converted to protective prostaglandin E3 that have been shown to slow tumor growth, inhibit angiogenesis, prevent proliferation, boost immune function and reduce inflammation.

They can be found in cold-water fish, such as salmon, tuna, cod, mackerel, herring, sardines, in flax, chia and hemp seeds, nuts, especially walnuts, grass-fed, pastured, free-range meats, poultry, eggs and dairy.

Although this may sound contradictory, we need both types, and many healthy food choices naturally contain both types of fatty acids. But some foods contain a much higher ratio of the pro-inflammatory fats (Omega 6's), and the standard American diet (aptly referred to as "SAD") contains very little anti-inflammatory (Omega 3's) fats. The average American consumes about 20 times more Omega 6's than Omega 3's.

We need to balance out this ratio, which ideally should be around 3:1. 3 parts Omega 6's to 1 part of Omega 3's. Best for us is a 1:1 ratio. The first step we can take toward achieving this balance, is to become aware of the type of fatty acid source in the food we are consuming on a regular basis.

Food journaling is a great way of actually seeing what we are feeding ourselves with; what you find in the journal may not necessarily correlate with what you think you may be eating.

Maintaining an Acid-Alkaline Balance

You may be wondering whether you should avoid acidic-tasting food like lemons or tomatoes as you may have heard that cancer cells thrive in an acidic environment. We need to look at the real underlying issue at stake, as it is not a matter of eating acidic-tasting foods that affect your blood and cell pH levels.

When we metabolize, or break down, food it is chemically oxidized ('burned') to form water, carbon dioxide and an inorganic compound. The nature of this inorganic compound that is left behind after the food is broken down determines whether the food is alkaline or acid-producing. Some refer to it as the "ash" left behind. If it contains more sodium, potassium or calcium, it's classed as an alkaline food. If it contains more sulphur, phosphate or chloride, it's classed as an acid food.

So, what happens to your body when it is too acidic? On the one hand, it stores excess acid in your fat cells, a factor which can contribute to a person having trouble losing weight. On the other hand, our body has a mechanism using mainly the lungs, kidneys and a mineral buffering system where it tries to balance out the excess acidity to restore equilibrium again.

Over time, this buffering system can drain our body of essential reserves of vital minerals and important enzymes. Minerals can get pulled from our bones, teeth, organs and tissues to compensate for an overly acidic body. This can lead to osteoporosis and loss of bone density. If there is simply too much acid for the body to handle, the blood will dump it in your tissues, leading to an accumulation of toxins. Your lymphatic system now tries to deal with it, but can end up dumping the excess it cannot deal with back into the blood.

So, why is this an issue? Blood carries oxygen to all your cells, ensuring healthy cells that can give you energy, and keep you healthy by being able to perform their specific function. Over-acidic blood causes a change in the electric charge of blood cells, causing them to clump up and not move around as freely, thus hindering the steady supply of oxygen throughout the body. Coupled with a lack of hydration, and most of us don't drink enough, oxygen does not get transported around as well. This is not good news for an anti-cancer environment.

Have you ever wondered why you sometimes wake up feeling groggy and overly sleepy even if you had sufficient hours of sleep, or why you are feeling overly thirsty? Think about it like this. We are made up of about 70% water. If that water is toxic due to an over-acidic environment, how much rejuvenating life force are we able to produce or absorb? That does not make for an anti-cancer environment.

That is why, for example, staying very hydrated during chemo is so vitally important to help reduce the toxic, acidic overload on your body.

If an overly acidic body drains our mineral reserves, this also has a direct effect other vital biochemical processes involving a myriad of enzymes.

Minerals play a key role in the production of enzymes. Enzymes not only play a part in renewing and repairing blood, tissues and organs, they are also a major player in proper digestion. We are dependent on a range of different digestive enzymes throughout the entire digestive process, starting in the mouth right down to your gut.

Here is the key: if we don't have enough digestive enzymes, the body will send its troops there to make more, and put a brake on the enzymes necessary for cell and tissue repair. There's a limit to everything.

Acidic food is not rich in enzymes, alkaline food is, in particular raw and living foods. Enzymes are destroyed by heat, and they are pH sensitive. Cooking above 118 degrees F (48 degrees C) destroys enzymes, and so does an acidic pH level. Processed foods are dead in that respect. That is why raw and living foods are so vitally important for us, as we supply our bodies with much-needed enzymes that give it a break from having to use its own reserves. Foods like fresh veggies, fruits, wheatgrass, nuts, seeds, grains, green juices and smoothies supply vital nutrients, minerals phytonutrients, fiber and above all, OXYGEN.

Remember, cancer cells don't like oxygen!

The Power of Plant Nutraceuticals

An overly acidic body has another problem - free radicals. When the body has to neutralize too much acidity, a result of this process is the creation of free radicals. These damage our cells, even though we can't eliminate all of them and actually need some free radicals to fight off bacteria and viruses, while also being part of normal cell metabolism. An excess of free radicals is the problem.

This is where anti-oxidants come to the rescue. A free radical is an unbalanced molecule that is lacking a part, an electron. It will go find one, and this "hunt and steal" phase can set off a cascade of reactions that can systematically damage your cells. Now anti-oxidants willingly give off an extra electron, thus calming down the free radical and diverting danger.

Where do we find an abundance of anti-oxidants? In raw, living plant foods!

Not only are they full of vital vitamins and minerals, but also so-called phytonutrients. Phytonutrients were discovered over the last 30 years or so, and there are 1000s of them, and many more still to be claimed. They are what protects plants from danger in nature, and for us they offer an amazing thing: an extra electron! They are what makes plant foods look vibrantly colorful and taste attractive.

Some common ones you may be familiar with include curcumin found in the bright orange turmeric root, sulforaphane in broccoli, cabbage and brussel sprouts, as well as resveratrol in blueberries, grapes and garlic. They are heat sensitive just like enzymes, therefore, eating "rainbow raw" should be an important part of your overall diet.

There are some anti-cancer diets that ask for eating raw only, including meats, to ensure a steady supply of raw, living enzymes. Others, call for a ratio of about 80% raw (in the form of vegetables) to 20% cooked foods, which is a way I like to encourage my clients to eat.

Ways of including raw foods into your diet include a variety of salads enhanced with as many raw vegetables as possible, a favorite way of getting my raw supply. With a sturdy, sharp grater and peeler you can turn any salad into a rich rainbow variety of living foods. Smoothies and fresh juices are another way of adding a dose of rainbow raw into your daily diet.

If you are now determined to avoid most acidic foods, you may want to think that over. A better ratio is preferable, remember everything in moderation, and balance is the key!

The standard American diet generally consists of an 80/20 ratio, 80 acidic/and 20 alkaline. An ideal ratio is 60-80 alkaline/ 20-40 acidic.

A word of caution - not all acidic foods are the same!

There are weak as well as strong acids; the weaker ones don't stress the body as much. Many of the healthy foods we ought to consume are more acidic, yet avoiding them could lead to potential nutritional deficiencies which defeat the purpose of adopting a cancer-fighting way of eating.

Here, I would like to make a note on the macrobiotic diet, which some say is an effective cancer-fighting diet. You may recall that I initially said that it is my view, based on my own experiences, as well as my research and interactions with respected colleagues in the functional medicine field, as well as working with all my clients, that there is no single anti-cancer diet that works for everyone.

A macrobiotic way of eating needs to be closely monitored as it can be too acidic, relying heavily on grains, a low fat intake, and mainly cooked food. Some may thrive on it, while others will actually feel a deterioration in health, overall.

Our bodies are unique, and regardless of the healthy style of eating we prefer to adopt, we need to monitor ourselves for possible nutrient deficiencies which could indicate potential digestion and subsequent absorption issues. A good rule of thumb is to include at least 60% raw, uncooked foods, a healthy essential fatty acid ratio, a great variety of fresh, colorful produce and an overall low glycemic way of eating to ensure steady blood sugar levels. This way we can actively support our body by truly nourishing it with real food, ensuring we create an internal environment that is inhospitable to cancer.

CHAPTER 4
STEP 2 – PART 1
REDUCE THE TOXIC EXPOSURE IN YOUR FOOD SUPPLY

"The dose makes the poison."
Paracelsus

When we look at our world today, it can be easy to become quite disillusioned about being able to give our body a fighting chance to withstand the seemingly constant bombardment of toxicity that has become part and parcel of our daily lives.

We are responsible for altering our external environment and introducing substances that can have a detrimental effect on our own, and our planet's health.

However, it is not my intention to have you walk away feeling pessimistic about being alive in the 21st Century! Our bodies can actually do a tremendous job eliminating toxic residue and adjusting to our surroundings, if we make smart decisions and try to help our bodies along the way.

Before you delve into this content-rich chapter, I want to assure you that you will find some balance moving forward as you weigh up the options of what you can easily change in your life, and what requires a more long-term approach. I, or rather we, as it involves the entire family, made a lot of adjustments either immediately, or over time. We certainly have areas to improve on, but we made the conscious decision at the time that what we were doing was sufficient, considering our way of life and our financial situation.

We made peace with our decisions and now continue to be grateful for what our modern life has to offer. Incessant worrying about whether or not everything we do is detrimental to our health is just as toxic as a physical-chemical itself.

We cannot live in a 100% toxin-free world, especially as many of the conveniences we have become accustomed to in our daily lives are based on technological developments that did not exist even a generation ago. In today's modern world we are subjected to man-made chemicals on a scale never seen before.

For us cancer warriors, we face a double burden if we have had our cancer cells bombarded with conventional treatments as they leave a hefty toxic footprint from which our bodies need some time, and outside help, to recover. This is a grey area, one where most conventional medical teams do not offer us any direct guidance, and we are left to our own devices to try to get ourselves back on track.

This is even more important when considering that an imbalanced environment causes cells to malfunction in the first place, and now we have contributed an additional toxic layer thanks to our treatments. Another reason why we need to be acutely aware of what receiving treatments actually means, mainly targeting cancer cells only for the most part. All the more crucial that we arm ourselves with strategies to help reduce the toxic burden, from the inside as well as the outside, so that our bodies can help fight cancer cells from within again, as they are supposed to.

Toxins and their residue bio-accumulate within our bodies, a little more each year. Taken one step further, these individual chemicals can react and interact with each other when brought together inside our tissues, adding to what is commonly referred to as the toxic load.

The extent this can create lasting damage varies; it can be an overwhelming load for some, but not others, and here's where our unique bodies come into play again.

For some of us, even a small toxic load can tip us over the edge. We may have been exposed to environmental toxins as children from the water supply we had access to, cigarette smoke from our parents, as in my case, our mother's, as well as our own, silver amalgam teeth fillings, or we may carry certain genetic mutations that reduce our body's ability to detox efficiently.

Signs of this can become evident when we, for example, suffer from constant allergies, while others around us don't, or we have sudden, severe reactions to that new sofa, a newly painted room or even a brand new car. Chances are high we are reacting to the "off-gassing" of volatile organic compounds (VOCs).

The Breast Cancer Prevention Partners (BCPP, formerly the Breast Cancer Fund), a non-profit, non-partisan organization dedicated to educating the public about cancer prevention, has this to say: "Laboratory studies have shown that organic solvents are direct mutagens and carcinogens, that is, these chemicals and their breakdown products can exert effects on genes and cells, influencing the rates of gene mutation and altering cell processes in ways that increase the risk of cancer" (Labreche, 1997). The BCPP has an entire library of research links to support their findings, and the link to their site can be found in the reference section later in this book.

As cancer conquerors, our underlying foundation is to ensure that we have a strong immune system capable of destroying any potentially cancerous cells. This is our overall goal, and needs to be the driving force behind every decision we take when it comes to our health.

So, how can we put this into action in a seemingly toxic world?

Let's start by looking at what a toxin is and the effect it can have on our body. A toxin is any substance that can interfere with the normal functioning of a cell, potentially leading it to malfunction. It is important to understand that even a healthy substance, if taken in excess, can be toxic to the body. Certain herbs, for example, if taken in very small dosages have a health-promoting effect, but if overdosed can be poisonous. Even water can be seen as a toxic substance if an excess amount is forced into a cell.

Synthetic or chemical toxins in our environment are harmful if they don't break down and begin to accumulate, affecting the normal functioning of the immediate, as well as neighboring surroundings. These are commonly referred to as POPs or "Persistent Organic Pollutants".

Before the 2nd world war, the substance of many common household products was based on plants. Even celluloid, a plastic-like material was derived from plants. After 1945 there was a huge shift in industrial production as the use of petrochemicals formed the basis of many household goods. These industries themselves produce tons of hazardous waste materials which end up polluting our environment, ultimately adding to the toxic body load.

The first public outcry in the US showing the link of environmental pollutants to a deterioration in health was Rachel Louise Carson's book *"The Silent Spring"* in the 1960's. It is a scientifically-based book that documented the detrimental effects that certain pesticides, in particular the spraying of DDT to kill mosquitoes, had on the environment, especially the bird population. The chemical industry was vehemently opposed to these findings, but it did lead to a revised national pesticide policy, a ban on the use of DDT and the creation of the EPA (Environmental Protection Agency) by President Nixon in 1970. Carson, a marine biologist and conservationist, suffered through repeated recurrences of breast cancer while researching and writing the book, eventually losing her battle soon after its release.

Still in the 1970's an MD by the name of Dr. Theron Randolph published a book called *"An Alternative Approach to Allergies,"* which was the first time that indoor air quality was linked to human health, referred to as the "sick building syndrome". Improper ventilation, the releasing of chemicals into the air (off-gassing) and molds from synthetic materials, wood smoke, radon gas and other factors have been shown to lead to DNA damage, birth defects, an increase in asthma as well as cancer rates.

So how does this become a problem?

Toxins are dangerous because they can affect the complex bio-chemical pathways in numerous ways. Raymond Francis, the author of *"Never Fear Cancer Again,"* sums it up concisely: toxins can immobilize enzymes necessary to regulate many bodily functions , mimic hormones and give false information to cells and genes, prevent cell to cell communication which can provide the wrong feedback and prevent the body from being able to self-regulate, damage DNA directly causing genetic mutations, react with DNA thereby changing the ways genes express themselves, and interfere with the transport of oxygen to cells.

From this list alone, it is clear what role toxins can play in creating an underlying, simmering environment in the body capable of enabling cancer cells to get a foothold.

In the 2008-2009 annual report of the President's Cancer Panel, which reports to the US President on the development and execution of the National Cancer Program set in motion by President Nixon in 1971, entitled *"Reducing Environmental Cancer Risk – What can we do now?"* it was reported that "the Panel was particularly concerned to find that the true burden of environmentally induced cancer has been grossly underestimated. With nearly 80,000 chemicals on the market in the United States, many of which are used by millions of Americans in their daily lives and are unstudied or understudied and largely unregulated, exposure to potential environmental carcinogens is widespread".

Although we are exposed to chemicals in minute quantities, we need to take into consideration that this exposure is relentless, and comes from many sources on a regular basis. We also know that these substances can bio-accumulate in our tissues.

The CDC (Center for Disease Control) conducts ongoing surveys in which they measure toxic residue in collected samples of blood and urine from the US population. The latest updates called The Updated Tables of January 2017, provide nationally representative biomonitoring data that has been available since the publication of the Fourth National Report on Human Exposure to Environmental Chemicals, 2009. It presents data for a total of 308 chemicals, which were found in the samples of most Americans tested. In particular, these six chemicals were found in almost every person sampled.

1. **PDEs (polybrominated diphenyl ethers)** – flame retardants added to most furniture, mattresses, carpeting and computers to reduce any potential fire hazard. These can accumulate in human fatty tissue and can damage the nervous system, liver and kidneys, sexual function. They can also cause brain disorders, thyroid problems and lead to cancer. The breast milk of women in the US has the highest levels of PDEs worldwide.

2. **BPA (bisphenol-A)** – found in plastic bottles and the plastic linings of cans. BPA is highly toxic even at very low dosages. It is a known endocrine disruptor; it can mimic our own hormones and unbalance our entire hormone system. Children are the most vulnerable. BPA can affect heart health, cause diabetes, liver damage, behavioral problems, asthma and obesity. It will weaken our kids' immune systems from the outset. CDC (Center for Disease Control) scientists found bisphenol-A in more than 90% of the urine samples representative of the U.S. population.

3. **PFOAs (per-fluoro-octanoic acid)** – is used in non-stick cookware, stain-resistant clothing, some food packaging and heat-resistant products. Studies link contamination to the liver and immune system dysfunction, reproductive problems as well as cancer.

4. **Acrylamide** – this is a chemical formed when frying, roasting, grilling or baking carbohydrate-rich foods at temperatures above 248 F (120 C). It has been found in foods such as bread, fried meats, French fries, chips, and coffee. Tobacco smoke is also a known culprit. Some studies link acrylamide to cancer.

5. **Mercury** – one of the most toxic heavy metals, is found in silver dental fillings, vaccinations and is also caused by eating contaminated fish. Mercury bio-accumulates and is passed to our babies. Studies have shown it to cause and promote cancer as it can prevent cell death (apoptosis), damage enzymes needed for oxygen respiration, and cause oxidative stress, which can lead to DNA damage. According to Francis in *"Never Fear Cancer Again"*, mercury can lower the T-cell count of our white blood cells, and it can reduce the capacity of our blood to carry oxygen by 50%. Studies have shown that removing mercury amalgam/silver fillings can result in a 50-300% increase in white T-Cell count.

Other heavy metals such as lead, cadmium and arsenic can also severely disrupt our body's biochemical reactions; it is highly advisable to check our mercury levels when considering a cancer-fighting lifestyle. This can be easily assessed and monitored with a lab test.

6. **MTBE (methyl tert-butyl ether)** – was added to gasoline years ago, and is no longer used today, yet it still shows up as one of the six chemicals found in almost all human urine and blood samples tested. Not just that, it is also still found in our US water supplies as well as in cigarette smoke, and has been shown to lead to neurological damage and reproductive disorders; it is also carcinogenic in high doses.

Ken Cook, founder and president of the Environmental Working Group (EWG), a non-profit, non-partisan organization that advocates for transparency and education when it comes to our lifestyle choices and government policies and regulations, testified before the US Senate Subcommittee on Superfunds, Toxins and Environmental Health in 2010, and stated that hundreds of chemicals were measured to be found in the blood of unborn babies still in the womb. (The link to this testimony can be found in the References section).

"As a result of the failed federal toxics program, we now have babies born pre-polluted in this country with a cocktail of over two hundred toxic chemicals already in their bloodstreams – many linked to some very serious health problems, including cancer, which are on the rise in the U.S."

This provides serious food for thought!

We can, nevertheless, do our part to consciously avoid or reduce our exposure to those toxins that can affect us in our immediate environment. With a little education, a willingness to sometimes ditch what seems most convenient, by being street smart, coupled with a healthy dose of skepticism regarding certain government regulations, we can choose what we allow ourselves to get into contact with on a daily basis.

We can become proactive toxin detectives and make sure we approach our modern conveniences with an "eyes-wide-open" approach to our food, our personal and cosmetic care and our home and household environment. Again, we have choices!

Let's take a closer look at the food offered in our multitude of supermarkets and what we end up stocking in our pantries.

We may be confident in believing that our food production in the US is regulated to ensure universal health and safety standards. Three agencies in the US are largely responsible for this. The USDA (US Dept of Agriculture), in particular the FSIS (Food Safety and Inspection Service) observes the natural states such as plants grown and animals raised, the FDA (Food & Drug Administration) tests the finished products, and the EPA (Environmental Protection Agency) monitors levels of chemical toxicity in food.

How safe is this regulated food? Is everything that is added to our processed food tested for safety levels, which would fall under the jurisdiction of both the FDA and EPA?

According to the FDA, a food additive is a substance that has no proven track record of safety and must, therefore, be tested for approval by the FDA before it is allowed to be added to the food. This is a good thing.

However, there are many ingredients in our food that are *not* defined as additives, but are generally recognized as safe (GRAS) because the FDA bases their approval on already published studies, or because it has been used in the food item for quite some time, thus making it exempt from approval. Many ingredients, which we will now look at have this GRAS status, and still many are not regulated at all. GRAS items are thus not tested, at least not on a regular basis by the FDA.

You may now ask yourself if these are substances to be found on our food labels. Some are, others aren't. It is staggering to see what goes into keeping our food fresh, edible and attractive looking, and what ends up in our bodies as a result.

I am going to highlight a few ingredients found in the items we generally recognize as our staple food. This book is not intended to provide you with an extensive list of ingredients to avoid. For that, I refer you to two outstanding publications by respected fellow colleagues Mira Dessey, NE and her book *"The Pantry Principle – How to read the label and understand what's really in your food"* and *"What the Fork are you Eating?"* by Stefanie Sacks.

I want to illustrate how we are often oblivious to what really goes into our food. There are many grey areas when it comes to whether or not ingredients are approved. Often the decision to use an ingredient or not, is based on whether there is sufficient evidence, either from studies or anecdotally based, to suggest that the ingredient is harmful to our health. It is easy to turn a blind eye and ignore the finer details. I want you to get a glimpse of why we ought to pay a lot more attention to what we choose to put in our and our family's mouths.

Standard questionable ingredients

To keep food from spoiling it has to be treated with **chemical preservatives** to prevent it from oxidizing and becoming moldy, to retain color, increase shelf life and prevent growth of pathogenic bacteria.

However, there is never any one single ingredient added to achieve this preservation. Promising research and food safety advocates are increasingly showing what can potentially happen when these different additives are combined and begin to react with each other or other substances inside your body.

Antimicrobials, such as **benzoates** (GRAS approved), when used in drinks that also contain ascorbic acid, can interact with each other to form **benzene,** which has been linked to cancer. The FDA has urged companies not to combine the two. This was initially ignored; a lawsuit in 2006 forced soft drink companies such as Coca-Cola & Pepsi Cola to reformulate their fruit-flavored drinks.

Potassium sorbate, another antimicrobial used to prevent the growth of mold, and also GRAS approved, can be found in cheese, baked goods, bread, tortillas, dried fruit, syrups and some wine. It has been shown to alter the DNA by being genotoxic to human lymphocytes, which are part of our white blood cells, and the basis of our immune system. Another study showed that if mixed with ascorbic acid (Vitamin C), which is found in many foods, it had the potential to change DNA structure.

Cured foods often have sodium nitrates and **sodium nitrites** added to preserve their pinkish color as well as prevent pathogenic bacterial growth. The problem isn't with the actual nitrates themselves as these are naturally occurring salts, but if combined in protein foods like lunch meats, they can react with other amino acids in protein foods forming combinations such as nitrosamines, which can lead to a cancer-causing potential. Incidentally, these occur naturally in fresh vegetables and when consumed nitrates turn to nitrites in saliva, however no harm is caused to the body.

BHA (Butylated Hydroxyanisole) is added to prevent fats from becoming rancid. Animal studies have shown a link to cancer, but no real human studies have yet been undertaken. It is still approved as GRAS by the FDA, but the US Department of Health & Human Services has stated that BHA can be anticipated to be classified as a human carcinogen.

Irradiation is a rather controversial subject as there is a long standing debate on whether it makes food radioactive or simply diminishes nutrient content. This process has been approved by the FDA, USDA, CDC & WHO (World Health Organization). The FDA requires the Radura Symbol on all radiated food, but not on foods that contain irradiated ingredients. A list of foods approved for irradiation in the US includes beef, pork, poultry, shellfish, fresh fruit and veggies, spices and seeds.

In their book "*Zapped! Irradiation & the Death of Food,*" Wenonah Hauter & Mark Worth illustrate how evidence exists that irradiated foods can lead to abnormal cell formation.

I have received seven weeks of radiation to my right upper torso. I see the long-lasting cell damage effects it has had, and am acutely aware of the potential for continued cell damage to escalate for years to come. I am not putting my trust in irradiated food as a source of nourishment of any kind.

Flavor Enhancers

The classic flavor enhancer, MSG – Monosodium Glutamate is GRAS approved. MSG is a derivative of the fairly common glutamic amino acid, which is naturally present in many foods such as cheeses and tomatoes, as well as in our bodies.

Originally extracted from a seaweed broth, today, MSG is produced by fermenting starch, sugar beets, sugar cane or molasses. The problem can arise from the denatured by-products of processed glutamic acid.

Although no real studies exist to prove it is unsafe, sufficient anecdotal evidence showed numerous health reactions in people sensitive to MSG. The FDA requires MSG to be listed as a separate ingredient on the packaging.

On their fda.gov website, it states that "*the FDA requires that foods containing added MSG list it in the ingredient panel on the packaging as monosodium glutamate. MSG occurs naturally in ingredients such as hydrolyzed vegetable protein, autolyzed yeast, hydrolyzed yeast, yeast extract, soy extracts, and protein isolate, as well as in tomatoes and cheeses. While the FDA requires that these products be listed on the ingredient panel, the agency does not require the label also to specify that they naturally contain MSG. However, foods with any ingredient that naturally contains MSG cannot claim "No MSG" or "No added MSG" on their packaging. MSG also cannot be listed as "spices and flavoring".*"

Food Coloring

Our grandmothers used natural, plant-based food coloring agents such as red and yellow beets or spinach greens; they did not need to offer food aflame with psychedelic vibrancies.

In 2010 The Center for Science in the Public Interest (CSPI) released their "Food Dyes: A Rainbow of Risks" report in which nine different dyes that are widely used in common foods are under the risk of cancer, hyperactivity and allergies spotlight.

The food industry uses over 15 million pounds of the dyes studied in our food supply each year. Three of the dyes carry known carcinogens, and four can cause serious allergic reactions in some consumers. New studies show that seven of these dyes contributed to cancer in lab animals, including brain and testicular tumors, colon cancer, and mutations.

"These synthetic chemicals do absolutely nothing to improve the nutritional quality or safety of foods, but trigger behavior problems in children and, possibly, cancer in anybody," said CSPI executive director Michael F. Jacobson.

James Huff, an associate at the National Toxicology Program commented, "Some dyes have caused cancers in animals, contain cancer-causing contaminants, or have been inadequately tested for cancer or other problems. Their continued use presents unnecessary risks to humans, especially young children. It's disappointing that the FDA has not addressed the toxic threat posed by food dyes."

Since 2009 the European Food Safety Authority (EFSA) has been reviewing the safety of all food additives approved for use by the EU up until that point in time, due to new scientific data becoming available. They began re-assessing 41 food colors and completed their evaluation in 2016. As a result of this study they lowered the Acceptable Daily Intake (ADI) for some food colors, and withdrew others from the market, due to their toxicity and subsequent effect on human safety.

In 2010 the EU ruled that all artificially dyed foods must have labels that warn of possible hyperactivity in children. As a result many manufacturers started using natural food coloring. A Strawberry Sundae in Europe gets its color from... yes, strawberries. In the USA this is Red No.40, which although has not yet been proven to cause cancer, has been shown to contain cancer-causing contaminants. Red#3 and Citrus Red#2 have been shown to cause cancer in lab rats.

Incidentally, most OTC (over the counter) NSAIDs (non-steroidal anti-inflammatory drugs) such as Advil, Motrin, Aleve and the like use artificial food coloring as a method of identification. Some diabetic, home-brands are dye-free, but they are often not readily available. In a 20-mile vicinity around my home, I can only get a dye-free Advil off the shelf at my local Walmart in their own diabetic store brand. Everywhere else, I need to specifically ask for a special order.

Artificial Sweeteners

A few words on artificial sweeteners. Consumers may happily use them as they have hardly any calories, and because of their level of sweetness less is needed, leaving the false impression that one is using very little sugar. The problem is that they are made from synthetic, chemical molecules our body cannot recognize.

They are used in most processed foods, and are found wherever the packaging says "light", "low or reduced" or "no-added sugar" or "zero calories". There are the potential health issues.

Saccharin (GRAS approved), found in Sweet n' Low, Sweet Twin, Nectar Sweet, has been around since 1879 when an accidental coal tar spill tasted sweet to a scientist. When, in the 1970's it was shown to possibly be related to bladder cancer in rats, the FDA tried to do its job and ban it. However this motion was overturned in a legal battle that involved the agricultural food giant Monsanto, who also happened to incidentally be the producer of Saccharin. (Sacks, S.)

An enraged public was 'drummed up' to view the ban as Big Government encroaching on the public interests against a backdrop of inconclusive scientific evidence that saccharin increased the risk for cancer in humans. As a result, a bill passed in 1977, stating that all saccharin products would carry a warning label. This health risk clause was revoked again in 2000 due to an apparent lack of sufficient scientific evidence deeming this labeling necessary.

Newer research suggests that saccharin can disrupt the diversity of bacterial strains we rely on in a healthy gut microbiome, potentially causing obesity. Where there is fuel, there is often fire, there is too much controversy about saccharin, and many other artificial ingredients, for me, as a consumer, to feel comfortable relying on a government agency to tell me it's generally recognized as safe.

We rely on scientific studies to establish baseline standards, and to confirm a condition based on measured actions with repeatable results. But let's not forget who often funds such research, and to what degree a scientific evaluation can be used to fully gauge the potential health risk. Perhaps the quantities deemed "safe" in a particular food item under question seems acceptable for some, what if you happen to fall into the category of extremely sensitive because your body struggles with proper methylation and detoxification, a fact you may not be aware of as traditional medicine does not analyze your body functions in that way.

Aspartame, found in NutraSweet, Equal and Sugar Twin, and most chewing gum, was linked in three independent studies to cancer in rodents, yet to date is still approved by the FDA.

The active ingredient in Splenda (GRAS approved), Sucralose is made by combining sucrose (table sugar) with chlorine. The problem with chlorine is two-fold. On its own, it is a highly toxic chemical, but its byproducts (organochlorines and dioxins) exacerbate the problem as they can interact with other toxins, compounding their detrimental effect on our health, and they are persistent in the environment, both inside and outside our body.

They do not break down easily, leading to the bio-accumulation I referred to earlier, mostly in the fatty tissue of humans – that is often a much more serious cause for concern. They are a known hormone disrupter and can mimic estrogen, having been documented by the EPA as also causing reproductive disturbances such as infertility and changes in fetal development in animals.

The impact chlorine has in terms of adding to our toxic burden calls for a much more in-depth analysis than is the scope of this book. Suffice it to say that the widespread use of chlorine in our municipal drinking water, the production of household items such as paper and paper towels as well as our personal care products, including most hygiene-related products such as sanitary pads, toilet and facial tissue paper, has led to its presence being felt in almost every household, even more so if you have a chlorinated pool. Whether or not this may be affecting your health, largely depends on your consistent levels of exposure and your body's ability to detox efficiently.

One more note on Splenda. Animal studies are increasingly showing that regular use of Splenda can lead to diminished levels of healthy gut bacteria, by as much as 50%, which in turn affects your overall immune system and nutrient absorption.

Sugar Alcohols, recognizable by the – ol ending such as erythritol, sorbitol, xylitol, mannitol, maltitol, lactitol, polyglycitol, and also isomalt, have made an increasing appearance in food products such as protein bars, ice creams, dietetic products and as sugar replacement in chewing gum that is not sweetened with either aspartame or ordinary cane sugar. These sweeteners are not made from either sugar or alcohol; they are a synthetic chemical creation that is not fully digested by the body and may potentially lead to a bloated feeling, excess gas or mild diarrhea.

A quick side note: both sugar alcohols and stevia (GRAS approved in refined form) are a low-glycemic sweetener; remember this is when your blood sugar does not spike after consumption.

A word of caution about a stevia-related product called Truvia. It is not stevia, but created from an isolated extract of the stevia leaf, in other words a processed, chemically derived product. Stevia in its true form has been used for hundreds of years in its country of origin, South America, and was even shown to have a blood sugar regulating effect in rats.

However, it was originally banned by the FDA based upon too little evidence of its safety. When the manufacturers of Truvia applied for FDA approval of Stevia, a GRAS status was granted for the use of the isolated extract in Truvia, even though it had not been fully-tested, as is required by the FDA, on both rats and mice. In addition, most studies have been sponsored by a Truvia manufacturing partner. (Dessey, M). There is grave concern that Truvia may lead to possible health issues as yet unknown. Stevia itself is still not FDA approved.

What about real sugar?

Harvested sugar cane is refined over various stages by filtering out the mineral-rich molasses to remove the color and further boiling finally delivers the white sugar sold in stores. **Sugar beets** are also processed in a similar way, leaving the end product devoid of any enriching minerals.

Liquid sugar on the other hand, most often comes from the starchy by-products of corn when it is processed and manufactured into things like cornmeal, corn flour and corn oil. Enzymes and acids are added to the corn grain to extract the sugar molecules.

The problem, of course, is the use of genetically modified corn as well as sugar beets, and the highly refined end product which is anything but a resemblance to real sugar. According to the Non-GMO Project, a non-governmental organization dedicated to educating consumers, sugar beets fall into the high-risk category, in 2010 over 90% of the sugar beet crop in the US was genetically modified. Where is this sugar used? In almost all conventionally bought processed goods many of us consume on a regular basis. More on GMOs a little further on.

Agave nectar is a liquid sweetener that often is the source of intense debate even among nutritionists. Although a low glycemic option, it is exceptionally high in fructose, which is a different sugar molecule mainly metabolized as fat, leading to potentially elevated triglyceride levels and insulin resistance if consumed in excess. It has become trendy, so production has increased to accommodate demand, but not always in a health-enhancing way. Agave nectar is highly processed and refined, leaving one to wonder why one would want to ditch one refined sugar form for another, as the final product is far removed from its original source.

Rather, reduce your overall sugar intake. Let's not replace one undesirable product with another but alter nothing about the daily quantity consumed.

Inside Kirstin's Pantry

In my opinion, the best form of sugar is what either is as close as possible to the real thing, or as minimally processed as possible.

I use a variety at home, used mainly for baking: pure maple syrup, honey, brown rice syrup, molasses, coconut palm sugar (made from the blossoms of coconut palm), turbinado sugar, sucranat sugar, muscovado sugar or organic cane sugar for baking. Although they have all been processed to get to their usable states, they are not as refined as white sugar and have at least some minerals left behind, although in minute quantities. They vary in crystal size, the level of stickiness and richness in flavor. I also have stevia in liquid form in my house, although I will admit that I am personally not a fan of its super sweet taste.

Bear in mind that it is still sugar. It has calories and it raises blood sugar levels and can lead to insulin resistance. Consuming moderate amounts is key, and while this can be vague and open to interpretation, I refer to a moderate amount as one that does not require daily consumption to satisfy a craving. A little should go a long way, and if it doesn't yet, we've got work to do!

Adjusting your taste buds to be happy with less sweet is a great way of keeping that sugar in its place, as an occasional treat. It takes 4-6 weeks to adjust your taste buds, so don't give up easily.

A few years ago I decided to take a "sugar-stock" and evaluate where I still exposed myself to too much sugar on a regular basis. I realized it was in my green tea, of which I have between 3 and 6 mugs a day. I had weaned myself off sweetened drinks, including fruit juices, but not when it came to my tea and the occasional coffee treat. Time to change that!

It was not easy at first, as green tea without sugar tasted vile. Yet, I knew what I had to do, to persevere and expose myself to sugarless green tea with the same consistency as always, even though I wanted to scrunch up my mouth with every sip.

It probably took me three weeks to become accustomed to the taste since I was so low-sugar overall anyway, but a miraculous thing happened. When I was preparing the morning green tea for both my husband and myself, he still got the dash of maple syrup. I accidentally swapped the mugs and took a sip of his, and ended up scrunching up my face at the super sweet taste! Only a few weeks previously that had been my standard agreeable level of sweetness that I enjoyed.

I now like the slightly bitter taste of my green tea, brewed at exactly two minutes, with the water no longer boiling. I can now fully enjoy the individual flavors of all my loose green teas, whereas previously, the sweetener dampened the true taste sensation. The same goes for my occasional cup of coffee (true cup size, not mug size). Different coffees have different flavors, and you will be amazed at how you will begin to evaluate what you are being served! Your taste buds can fully develop once they are not numbed by same-sweet all the time.

Trans Fats and Hydrogenated Oils

I talked about the dangers of these in more detail in a previous chapter, here I simply wish to highlight again that these are chemically derived products that turn liquid oils into solid fats by adding hydrogen.

Our bodies are not meant to digest this type of fat as it damages the consistency of our cell membranes. There is also a definite link to trans fats raising certain cholesterol levels (LDL – bad cholesterol). In 2006 Harvard University published a study showing that trans fats can lead to heart disease. It took another decade, but to date, trans fats now need to be labeled separately on Nutrition Labels, but only if the food item contains more than 0.5g. Anything below that amount need not be labeled. Another reason why it is imperative that you limit your exposure to processed foods as far as possible.

Inside Kirstin's Pantry

I have made two choices: I limit my exposure to processed foods to only about 5% and I use fats and oils wisely. My pantry is stocked with organic extra-virgin olive oil, organic ghee (clarified butter), coconut oil (unrefined if possible) and real pastured butter for cooking and baking. Certain oils I keep as flavor enhancers in salads and on top of already roasted vegetables; these include sesame oil, toasted sesame oil, walnut oil, avocado oil, and flax seed oil. This may seem a lot, but I like variety when it comes to taste infusions, and some of the oils above come in small bottles.

Pesticides

In the US, the usage of pesticides, such as insecticides, herbicides, fungicides and rodenticides, exceeds 1 billion pounds on average each year, worldwide it is over 5 billion pounds.

What are the implications of these staggering statistics for us, the consumer? Are the effects this has in any way measured or regulated? There is a governmental regulatory program in place set up in 1991 by the USDA, called the Pesticide Data Program (PDP). The PDP's role is to collect pesticide residue data on mostly fruits and vegetables. This data is used by the EPA to establish its dietary risk assessment and pesticide registration process, by the FDA to refine sampling for enforcement of tolerances; by the Foreign Agricultural Service to support export of U.S. commodities in a competitive global market and by the Economic Research Service to evaluate pesticide alternatives; as well as by the public sector to address food safety issues.

The 2015 PDP annual summary report states that "over 99% of

the samples tested (10,187 with 96% from fresh and processed fruit and vegetables) had residues well below the tolerances established by the EPA".

In 2012 a French farmer sued one of the biggest agricultural giants and one of the leading contributors to pesticide contamination in the world, Monsanto, for not disclosing potential health hazard of pesticide weed killer Lasso after experiencing neurological problems, memory loss, headaches and stammering when exposed to this chemical in 2004.

How can there be this discrepancy? The problem is that the producers of chemicals used on food crops and in livestock farms are often in charge of testing them for use on food. The manufacturing industry and government regulatory agencies seem to rotate staff. Sad, but true. It requires us to be even more vigilant about whom we can trust when it comes to food and environmental safety regulations.

The Environmental Working Group (EWG), a leading not-for-profit environmental health, research and advocacy group, is a great resource for reliable, evidence-based information. Their evidence-based shopper's guide to pesticide residue, called 'The Dirty Dozen', lists those foods that show the highest pesticide retention when exposed to certain chemicals. These include apples, strawberries, grapes, peaches, imported nectarines, celery, spinach, sweet bell peppers, cucumbers, potatoes, cherry tomatoes, hot peppers.

They also publish a 'Clean Fifteen' list, which states which foods are acceptable; this is useful to know, particularly if your budget dictates that you only buy organic selectively.

Antibiotics

When antibiotics were first introduced, they bridged a gap in medical intervention and helped save millions of lives. They still play a key role in fighting off highly infectious diseases today.

However, the problem is an overexposure and subsequent resistance as well as toxicity due not to our own use, but consuming it in our food. Daily prophylactic use is common in factory farms to cover up sub-standard and unhygienic living conditions for most conventional livestock. I won't go into detail here, watch the movie "Food Inc" and you will get a taste of what our conventionally-raised animals in the US go through so that we can pay discounted prices at the supermarkets.

According to the EWG, almost 70% of antibiotics sold in the US goes to food-producing animals. The FDA stated in its 2012 Summary Report on Antimicrobials Sold and Distributed for use in Food-Producing Animals that the amount of antibiotics sold to farmers and ranchers for use in animals raised for meat grew between 16% and 37% percent from 2009 to 2012, depending on the class of drugs.

How can you protect yourself and ensure that you get clean meat? Look out for 3rd party verification seals of approval from NGO's (non-governmental organizations) Two common ones are the **AWA (Animal Welfare Approved)** or **CertifiedHumane.org**. They also offer resources online to help you find a trusted local farm to buy from. **Localharvest.com** is another great reference point to start off with.

Many local farms do not necessarily have these seals, but check them out anyway. Ask questions on how they keep their animals and what measures they take when they get sick. If livestock gets sick some antibiotic use is warranted, but only under closely monitored conditions and those animals will be kept apart, until fully recovered and anti-biotic-residue free. Your local farms are part of your community; they are just as invested in having a harmonious relationship with it as you are. You have a right to transparent answers if you want to support them.

We buy our fresh produce, eggs and most meat from a local farm where we have purchased CSA (community-supported agriculture) shares. They offer free range, grass-fed meats (beef, lamb, buffalo, pork) and poultry and eggs from pastured, happily clucking chickens. The cows come to the fence when you approach. The pigs can be pigs, rummaging around and oinking and grunting with each other. You can see how and with what methods they grow all the produce. The same farm workers appear year-after-year, and you interact with owner, farmers and laborers. There is full transparency and the personal pride is evident. The quality of this real, fresh food is superb, and all this an hour outside New York City!

Hormones

The use of hormones was first approved for use in the 1950s. In the US there are six different types, which are used in cattle. One of the most publically known is the use of the growth hormone rBGH (recombinant bovine growth hormone) on milk-producing cattle to stimulate accelerated maturity and increased milk production, and the potentially resulting cell growth promoting effects it has especially when it combines with another, naturally occurring hormone IGF (insulin-like growth factor).

The FDA considers rBGH safe, like all other hormones, but for us cancer warriors, this is an additional burden to an already hormonal drink. Having additional growth stimulating hormones is not a great idea. Bear in mind that the European Union, a mutually supportive conglomeration of 28 countries, banned hormone use in cattle, and rejected the import of hormone-treated beef way back in the 1980's. Here in the US, at the date of this publication, they are still considered safe.

As mentioned above, the same 3rd party verification groups AWA (Animal Welfare Approved) and CertifiedHumane.org offer their seals of approval, and give us an indication of whether a food source can be trusted or not.

GMOs (Genetically Modified Organisms)

The problem with GMOs is that we simply do not know the full extent that exposing ourselves to these chemically altered molecules has on our long term health, potentially affecting us as well as our children. In a way it is like being a part of a science experiment for years, just that we are not being monitored as you would under an official clinical trial. GMOs have never been tested for their safety; they have only been presumed safe, which is not the same thing.

Approximately 92% of US corn crop is genetically modified (Center for Food Safety). Soybeans and cotton each stand at 94%. As stated on their website, the Center for Food Safety currently estimates that about 75% of processed foods on US supermarket shelves contain some genetically modified ingredients.

GM herbicide-tolerant crops allow farmers to use specific herbicides that will kill weeds without harming their crop. Herbicide

residue still sticks and gets absorbed, even if the plar
tinues growing. Unfortunately, the supplier of the
and in turn, the pesticides to be used on that crop,
and the same company; it has a vested interest in the success of
both, but possibly at the expense of the health of the consumer
as well as the environment.

One of the balance-interrupting results are often so-called
super weeds that have become pesticide-resistant. As a result,
farmers have to use even more toxic pesticides, and so the toxic
cycle continues.

I have to shine the spotlight on glyphosate, the active ingredient in Monsanto's widely used Roundup weed killer, widely used
commercially and in households. Substantial evidence exists
linking severe health consequences to plants, animals and even
humans exposed to glyphosate. Studies have shown it is a known
endocrine disrupter, resulting in hormonal imbalances that can
affect healthy estrogen metabolism. Today, most breast cancers are estrogen positive. Glyphosate has been shown to cause
breast cancer growth through estrogen receptors in cancer cells.

Isn't it a wise decision then to figure out an alternative source
for killing your garden pathway weeds? I too was one of the igno-
ramuses and used Roundup when we initially arrived in the US,
when having a perfectly manicured property was still a priority. It
seems ridiculous now, but we all mature through our life's challenges, and hopefully, wake up and become aware of just what
we are doing to ourselves when we place modern conveniences
and superficial prettiness over critical awareness, a healthy dose
of skepticism and ultimately, our life span.

I remember being hugely impressed with the size and impeccably proportioned fresh produce when I first set foot in the US. And stuffing our first mega-turkey for our first Thanksgiving, having obtained it for free by collecting supermarket vouchers in the previous months. I was ignorant of the facts, and blinded by the trust we place in the system, assuming it does no harm. I grew up never doubting the authenticity of the food we buy from shops.

The cancer statistics nowadays paint a different picture, and we are each responsible for educating ourselves and adjusting our lifestyle choices accordingly. And if you think this way of life is too expensive, I want to share my simple, but powerful resolution: my health is my most important asset! It can be done without having to break the monthly budget, if we are willing to take a close look at how we allocate our monthly expenses. There is always a way if we place our health first. We just need to want to do it, and be willing to change our priorities.

Which label can we trust?

As much as I like my local farmer, I simply don't get everything I need from him; I also need some convenience and essential items in my pantry. This is where smart label knowledge comes in handy to help keep us informed about the products we buy.

The NON-GMO Project (www.nongmoproject.org) is a great resource for understanding how we can protect ourselves from GMO-food. They offer a non-GMO shopping guide, which is available as an App for your smart phone.

If you are wondering how long it is going to take you to shop from now on, rest assured, this will get a lot easier once you become accustomed to it.

It will take a bit of extra time in the beginning if you are not used to label shopping, but you will soon figure out what is your best bet, and then this new way of shopping will become routine before you know it!

Our water supply

Having access to clean water is one of the things that distinguishes a 1st world from a 3rd world country, as many highly contagious diseases are water-borne. Our 1st world "clean" water has nevertheless become a contributing factor to the underlying causes of our chronic disease explosion. Volatile Organic compounds (VOCs) as well as other by-products of chlorination can be classified as contaminants that have been shown to be carcinogenic. Often city water is tainted by heavy metals and radioactive materials.

Drinking bottled water may not necessarily be safer. Components of the plastic can leach into the water when exposed to heat (for example in a hot car) creating xenoestrogens inside our body that disrupt our normal hormonal metabolism, possibly contributing to a higher than normal estrogen level which our body struggles to get rid of. We need to be aware of this, as those of us post-breast cancer with hormone positive receptors need to become very savvy about all the areas where we are exposed to excess estrogen.

The easiest way to have access to clean, safe water, is to avoid plastic bottled water and use your own glass or BPA-free water bottles filled with filtered water from your home.

Have your water supply tested before you take any measures, so that you know exactly where you stand.

When choosing a water testing method or kit, make sure you understand what exactly is being tested. Local municipalities are usually equipped to test well water for free. Public water suppliers have their own tests and you can enquire what elements they include in their testing to meet regulatory requirements.

If you have never done this, knowing what to ask for may seem daunting. We chose an independent water test company to test our well water at home as we wanted to know absolutely everything, ranging from a wide range of contaminants to personal body care products and pharmaceutical residues, even though one would assume well water is free of these. They usually offer different test kits at different price ranges, the most comprehensive test being around the $250-300 price range. They also list everything they will test so you can make an informed decision.

Well water differs greatly to public/city water, which almost always has chlorine and fluoride added.

I have explained the issue with chlorine in a previous chapter, namely that it can react with other organic compounds and that the resulting organo-chloride compounds can be carcinogenic. Fluoride was introduced into the US water system to prevent tooth decay even though at the time, it was already a known carcinogen. The chief chemist at the National Cancer Institute, Dr. Dean Berk, has been famously quoted when he testified before Congress that "In point of fact, fluoride causes more human cancer death, and causes it faster than any other chemical."

Fluoride changes our enzymes, causing them to mutate or even become ineffective, leading to DNA damage and affecting the immune system and our aging process. It has also been shown that cities that use fluoridated water have more, not less tooth decay, as fluoride has been shown to leach vital minerals from bones and teeth.

The FDA has never approved adding fluoride to drinking water! It is still used in public water sanitation today. It is also offered in dentists' offices as part of the routine bi-annual teeth cleaning procedure, and if it is known that you live in a non-fluoridated area your kids may well get fluoride supplements prescribed. You have a right to refuse this, or simply go to a different dentist.

I grew up on fluoride tablets. I did not get them in South Africa, but when we moved to Germany in the late 1970's my friend was using them and I decided to do the same, without even figuring out whether I needed them and what they were for. We thought they were a vitamin supplement... I remembered this when I had my own kids and spoke to my dentist about it, who at least educated me about whether or not our municipal water had it added, and that in that case they did not need to supplement with it! I trusted the system, and saw no need to question it at the time. I now know better!

Various types of water filtration systems are available. One of the most effective ones at removing chemical toxins and disease-causing organisms is a reverse osmosis system, which uses a semipermeable membrane and water pressure to filter impurities out from your tap water. It comes in various sizes and offers a whole house system too so you can be assured that even your shower water is cleared of contaminants. It is an expensive option though, needs regular servicing and wastes a lot of water, using about 3 gallons of water for every gallon of filtered water.

The activated carbon filters are a great cost-effective option, and remove not only bad taste and odor, but also certain volatile chemicals, pesticide residue, some heavy metals like lead and copper, and chlorine. They don't filter out any fluoride or disease-causing organisms. Brands vary in terms of how many contaminants they effectively filter out, so do your research and understand why you need to filter your water in the first place. Although, to our surprise, our well water tested clean, we still use a Brita pitcher filter as it enhances the taste of our water.

I would like to end this discourse on environmental toxins with a promising regulatory development. In June 2016, a new law passed, the Frank R. Lautenberg Chemical Safety for the 21st Century Act, which, according to the EPA, addresses fundamental flaws in the Toxic Substances Control Act (TSCA) that have, for nearly 40 years, limited EPAs ability to protect the public from dangerous chemicals. The EPA views the law as a major victory for chemical safety, public health and the environment – particularly the mandatory duty to evaluate chemicals and the new risk-based safety standard." With the current political developments in the US in 2017, I truly and sincerely hope this health-enhancing initiative will still be supported in the coming years.

*Would a basic **CLEAN PRODUCTS Cheat Sheet** be helpful? I have one for you to download right now! Click here if you are reading a digital book version*

http://www.kirstinscancercare.com/clean-products-cheat-sheet/

or find it at

www.kirstinscancercare.com/awesomebookbonuses/

CHAPTER 5
STEP 2 – PART 2
REDUCE THE TOXIC EXPOSURE
IN YOUR HOME

"Let's clean up our environment. Let's clean up our bodies, but most importantly, let's not permit our babies of the future to be polluted before they are even born."
Louise Slaughter

Cleansing our cosmetics and personal care products

"But we don't eat or drink them, how can they be a problem" is sometimes a common reaction when I mention the fact that many of our personal beauty and skin care products contain harmful chemicals. Consider the fact that our skin is our largest organ, and it is permeable. It absorbs everything, and as we have learnt, certain substances can bio-accumulate in our tissues.

In their book *"The Safe Shopper's Bible,"* Dr. Samuel Epstein, Professor Emeritus of Environmental & Occupational Health at the University of Illinois' School of Public Health, and Chairman of the Cancer Prevention Coalition, and David Steinman, environmentalist and health consumer advocate, both internationally recognized authors on the avoidable causes of cancer, claimed back in 1995 that no cosmetics company warns consumers that their products may contain several common cosmetic ingredients that are themselves possibly carcinogenic, or that their contaminants may be carcinogenic precursors.

Fast forward twenty years, and the consumer is still left to their own investigative devices to figure out which products are safest to use.

Several studies have linked certain ingredients in shampoos, hair dyes, body lotions and cosmetics to a higher incidence of various types of cancer, especially if these people are prone to having a compromised detoxification system, meaning they can eliminate the toxic residue more slowly, and less efficiently, than others. This is where our bio-individuality comes into play again – we are not all the same, and may not know where we are on the detox-ability spectrum. If we indeed react to a particular product consider it a direct and obvious warning from our bodies.

It is usually a lot more subtle – we do not react at all, oblivious to the fact that we are adding to our toxic burden a tiny molecule at a time.

I have the challenging task of guiding my teenage daughter through the perils of mass advertising and the unwillingness so typical of this age to accept "unpopular" facts that would separate her from doing what everyone else is doing, despite growing up in a "clean" household.

According to the Breast Cancer Prevention Partners (formerly the Breast Cancer Fund), the cosmetics industry uses thousands of synthetic chemicals that are simultaneously applied in manufacturing processes to clean industrial equipment, stabilize pesticides and grease gears. The cosmetics industry to date remains largely unregulated at a federal level, resulting in an accumulation of chemicals that have been linked to chronic diseases like cancer as well as infertility and birth defects. A correlation can be made with the increase in introducing untested chemicals and the rise in breast cancer diagnoses.

Here is a basic list of some commonly used ingredients to avoid in the following products we all use on a daily basis, based on information found on the website of the Breast Cancer Prevention Partners (www.bcpp.org).

It is by no means a complete list of ingredients to avoid; it serves mainly as a starting point for you to become aware of why it is important that we become vigilant when making purchasing decisions that could potentially expose us to an accumulation of carcinogenic toxins that add to our body load and could tip us over the edge.

Shampoos & Conditioners, Creams and Body Lotions, Hair Spray, Toothpaste and Mouth Washes, Soaps, Hair Dye, Antiperspirants, Deodorants, After Shave Lotions, Lipstick, Lipliner, Eye Shadow and Eyeliners with:

- **triclosan** (classified as a pesticide to prevent bacterial growth and mold, it interferes with hormones production in particular the thyroid and breast development)

- **1,4-dioxane** (derived from petroleum, used to produce

the sudsing effect, ranked by International Agency for Research on Cancer (IARC) as a possible carcinogen, and by the National Toxicology Program (NTP) as a reasonably anticipated carcinogen. Sodium lauryl sulfate may be contaminated with 1,4-dioxane, thus avoiding SLS is a preferred choice.

- **parabens** (preservatives and anti-microbial agent, they have been found in samples of breast cancer tumor biopsies)

- **phthalates** (used in fragrances and nail polish, have been found to mimic estrogen and linked to early puberty in girls)

- **ethylene oxide** (used to counteract the harshness of sudsing agents and also to sterilize surgical instruments, it is a classified human carcinogen and is one of 51 chemicals that the National Toxicology Program (NTP) identifies as mammary carcinogens in animals)

- **1,3-butadiene** (in shaving creams, sprays, sunscreen, make-up foundation and anti-fungal treatments has been shown to increase mammary tumors in rats)

- **Polycyclic Aromatic Hydrocarbons (PAHs)** (naturally in coal, crude oil and gasoline are sometimes added to cosmetics and shampoos and have been linked to an increased breast cancer risk)

- **Lead** (may be found in over 650 cosmetic products, such as sunscreens, foundation, nail colors, lipsticks and whitening toothpaste, it is a proven neurotoxin, connected to learning and behavioral problems miscarriage, reduced fertility and delays in the onset of puberty in girls)

Another great resource is the EWG's Skin Deep Cosmetics Database which allows you to compare existing cosmetic and beauty care products ranked by level of contamination, based on information disclosed by the manufacturer. Especially the sunscreen guide, reviewed annually, is a very useful resource to have on hand to help you, the consumer, sift through all the conflicting information and make an informed purchasing choice.

Cleansing our home environment

Indoor pollution is sneaky – it exposes us to risks in the very environment we would like to consider safe. Materials used in construction, decoration and furnishings can off-gas certain VOCs, volatile organic compounds, as mentioned earlier in this chapter.

Most of them are odorless and off-gassed from products such as manufactured wood particle products, permanent press clothing, upholstery and drapes. We are also exposed to radiation, electromagnetic fields, molds and mildew, asbestos, heavy metals and gasses from combustion appliances like our heating systems, our technological gadgets such as TVs, computers, Wi-Fi, cell phones and most electrical appliances.

Formaldehyde, one of the odorless ones, is worthy of special attention. Used in pressed-wood products, glues and adhesives, permanent-press fabrics, paper product coatings, and certain insulation materials, as well as industrial fungicides and disinfectants, according to the National Cancer Institute (NCI), the EPA originally classified formaldehyde as a probable human carcinogen under conditions of unusually high or prolonged exposure. Since then, human studies have linked formaldehyde exposure with certain types of cancer. The International Agency for Research on Cancer (IARC) classifies formaldehyde as a human carcinogen, and it was first listed in the National Toxicology Report as a known human carcinogen in the Second Annual Report on Carcinogens in 1981.

How can you protect yourself considering you cannot move to a deserted island? Here's what you can do for starters:

- Ventilate – well and often! Especially if you buy a new car, new furniture, new carpets or paint. Open your windows and let that fresh air radiate through your home or car as often as possible.

- Make sure your heating system, chimneys and vents work properly, have them serviced regularly. Avoid exposure to tobacco smoke and scented candles.

- Use natural cleaning supplies as most conventional ones emit strong VOCs (some leading brands contain phenols and 1,4-dioxane (see above) or the strong pungent odor of bleach (chlorine).

- Wash your new clothes before wearing them – that is not a clean clothes smell, but a chemical cocktail smell.

- Consult the **EWG's Guide to Healthy Cleaning** that allows you to rank and compare common leading brands, including so-called "green" and organic ones (see Resources section).

- Make your own household cleaners! Get back to the roots of cleaning and use baking soda, hydrogen peroxide, distilled white vinegar, lemon juice and some essential oils. For example, I use only vinegar and Dr.

Bronner's Pure Castille soap (with essential oils) in water as our floor cleaner.

Electro pollution

Our immediate and extended environment is increasingly becoming polluted with a different, more invisible force called electro pollution. Ever since the advent of electricity we have been exposed to a degree of electric smog, so this form of exposure, and the possible effects it can have on our health, is nothing new. The earth itself exudes electromagnetic waves which can affect some of us detrimentally. The rate at which this exposure is exacerbated by our ever increasing accumulating of technological devices, however, is new.

In today's age it is impossible to think of our world without our interconnectedness through cell phones, tablets, and computers. EMFs (electro-magnetic fields) are not just emitted from these modern devices. We need to understand that these force fields surround anything that is powered by electricity, including every single electrical appliance in your home and also any outlet and electrical cable in the wall of your house.

A distinction needs to be made whether or not a person has what is called electromagnetic hypersensitivity (EHS), which causes a much more severe reaction to exposure at almost any level, even just the normal electrical wiring in your house. People with EHS can experience symptoms such as pressure headaches, tingling and burning in body parts and often suffer from chronic insomnia.

Larry Burk, MD, explains in his book "*Let Magic Happen – Adventures in Healing with a Holistic Radiologist,*" how he was trying to get to the root cause of his restless leg syndrome and persistent insomnia that seemed to defy all other holistic remedies he had been trying over a number of years. After an EMF evaluation of his house, he found a miraculous improvement in his quality of sleep and physical symptoms once he cut off the circuit breaker to his bedroom at night to decrease the body voltage from the wiring in the walls.

Stray radio frequencies (RF) coming from cordless phones and other wireless devices can also lead to constant radiation exposure. All wireless devices receive signals from the nearest base tower, even if not in use.

Over the last decade, the radical expansion of the wireless telecom industry has seen a steady increase in data linking cell phone use to brain tumors (Burk). Devra Davis, PhD is a leading pioneer in environmental toxicology. In 2007, Davis founded the non-profit Environmental Health Trust to provide basic research and education about environmental health hazards and to promote constructive policies locally, nationally and internationally. In their "Show me the Science" section on their website (see Resources section) you can find a host of peer-reviewed research studies linking EMF exposure to cancer and other chronic diseases.

In her book "*Disconnect: The Truth About Cell Phone Radiation, What the Industry is Doing to Hide It, and How To Protect Your Family,*" *(2011),* Davis documents how epidemiologist George Carlo, hired by the telecom industry to originally research and ascertain the safety of wireless technology, inadvertently found out that EMF exposure similar to what we receive from cell phones led to DNA damage and the inability of cells to repair themselves in animals. His studies were suppressed by the industry at the time, and were never published. He nevertheless, went public with his findings of the inadequacy of research sponsored by the cell phone industry (Burk).

An increasing amount of studies are slowly mounting that EMFs can lead to disruptions in the body's delicate biochemical, neurological and endocrine systems, ultimately affecting our cell health and the inability to repair DNA damage, which can possibly lead to cancer. For example, thermal images of brains after cell phone use are alarming and showcase just how much inflammation a single cell phone conversation can cause.

The International Agency for the Research on Cancer (IARC) released a report in 2011 in which they classified RF-EMF as a Group 2B carcinogen, meaning that there is a possibility that these are carcinogenic to humans. Further research showed that EMFs could act as a co-promoter in the presence of other carcinogens. Plainly stated, if the body burden is already loaded with carcinogenic exposure, adding EMFs can tip the scale, allowing for cancer growth to develop.

Here are a few things you can implement right away to reduce the effects EMFs may be having on your and your family's bodies:

- Limit or avoid any electrical appliances in your bedroom. At home, we only have our lamps. Our alarm clock is old-fashioned and battery-operated. We do not have a TV, nor do we keep cell phones or any other device in the bedroom. If you have to have a cell phone present, keep it far away from the head area and in airplane mode or even turned off.

- Turn off whole house wireless at night.

- Turn off as many appliances as you can, even unplug them.

- When speaking on your phone, use earphones or the speaker function rather than holding your cell phone to your ear.

- Try not to expose yourself to a computer screen right up to bedtime.

When I was first diagnosed with breast cancer, we lived in Munich, Germany where one usually lives in close proximity to one's neighbors, often in attached housing. I wanted to know whether I had been exposed to any "dirty" electricity," which are frequencies generated from all electronic devices in the nearby vicinity, in particular when I was asleep.

We hired an EMF measuring consultant, who was certified by the Institut für Baubiologie und Nachhaltigkeit, an industry-independent, non-governmental organization that advises on a harmonious relationship between humans and their environment. An equivalent organization in the US is the International Institute for Bau-Biologie and Ecology.

She arrived with her measuring equipment, and went to task analyzing, scanning, measuring and bleeping her way through our house, my ever-skeptical engineer husband in tow. The result was us purchasing a grounding bed pad for my side of the bed to reduce the higher voltage she found underneath my mattress, but nowhere else in the house. This was as a result of natural radiation emitted by the earth and not so much the accumulation of dirty electricity.

She found the wireless router from the attached house next door, and a host of other electrical appliances, but none were in excessive amounts, at least the needle did not shoot into the red section of her measuring device. My hubby did not fail to ask by how much her readings were affected by the EMFs emitted from her own equipment...

I cannot confirm whether this was a contributing cause to my cancer. A multitude of causative effects combine when it comes to why we each get our very individual cancers. Nevertheless, to this day, my grounding pad is still attached beneath my bed.

I have become very conscious about how I use my cell phone, and can feel the effect it has if I hold it close to my ear during a conversation. That feeling of an internal buzz is enough to set me straight in the event I have to take a call and do not have my ear phones ready or am unable to place the call on speaker. I either do not pick up the call, resorting to phoning back once I am set up, or I simply ask the caller to give me a moment to get ready. We do not have to feel strange about doing this; let's start a universal trend and before long it will become the norm.

I also practice **Earthing.** Ancient wisdom has taught us that an intricate system of energetic meridian lines run through and interconnect our body with its own parts, but also with our universal energy flow. This is what we tap into when doing acupuncture or applying acupressure to certain zones on our body. Those that conglomerate in our feet have a special role as they allow for a free flow of energy to connect us with the grounding energy field of our earth. As we wear shoes with rubber soles most of the time, we interrupt that flow. This life force energy is known in many cultures by different names, such as prana, qui, ki, Holy Spirit and universal energy.

In their book *"Earthing – The Most Important Health Discovery Ever"* (*2nd edition 2014*) by retired cable TV executive Clinton Ober and integrative cardiologist Dr. Stephen T Sinatra M.D. they go a step further and hypothesize that this earth connection has another healing benefit. Being connected to the negatively charged earth allows for an abundance of electrons to neutralize free radicals which are positively charged. This gives the body an antioxidant boost, exactly what a cancer-fighting body needs!

We can earth ourselves simply by taking off our shoes and connecting with mother nature bare feet, when the season allows. There are numerous ways in which you can help yourself become grounded, again. *"Getting Grounded: For Health and Healing,"* by Michael Hetherington (2015) is a great book for beginners; it is also a quick read.

For starters, I simply want you to become aware of the fact that we are connected with the earth and that this can contribute to our overall healing success.

There are a myriad of EMF protection devices on the market these days, and once again, I make reference to my skeptical scientific-minded husband, who keeps me grounded when it comes to the next best toy in the EMF protector world.

In 2015 a new EWG analysis of data submitted to the Federal Communications Commission showed that some smart phone cases, although not an official EMF protection device, actually intensify the radiation to the head. Poorly designed cell phone cases can partially block a phone's antenna, making the device work harder to transmit signals, thus exposing the user to more increased radiation.

I find the BioGeometry approach postulated by Dr. Ibrahim Karim to energy balancing and radiation exposure reduction, a useful and credible source of information and practical personal gadgets.

On their website they explain that "BioGeometry® is the patented science of using the energy principles of shape to qualitatively balance biological energy systems and harmonize their interactions with the environment".

They offer a number of products as solutions to balance disruptive personal and environmental energy sources. They approach EMF protection from cell phones by focusing on harmonizing the phone's EMF energy field with the body's own energy field, rather than blocking off transmission. Their principle is based on the ancient science of using geometrical patterns and shapes and the energy resonance they emit to balance energy patterns within organs of the body, a similar concept to that of Chinese energy meridians.

Why don't we all get sick, since we are all exposed to these conditions in today's developed world? Some of us have a higher toxic burden than others, and because of varying exposures in our work, school and home environments, nutritional deficiencies and our body's inability to detoxify properly or pre-existing genetic mutations, this can lead to some bodies not being able to cope with their particular body burden.

The good news is that once our particular body burden is identified, we can actively work on reversing this and restoring our cellular health again. Certain functional lab tests can help us identify our own particular burden, and then through a systematic and bio-individual approach slowly work on detoxifying our internal environment.

I strongly caution against a DIY approach as such a detox regimen needs to be closely monitored and constantly adjusted. Releasing toxins from our cells and ensuring they can be cleared through our own detox and methylation pathways can lead to severe side effects themselves that we need to understand and interpret correctly.

Working from the inside needs to be supported by us making the necessary adjustments to our outside environment as much as is reasonable. It is easy to get lost in a maze of "should do's," but with a systematic approach here too, a solution that works for you and your family can easily be identified.

A final note about consumer protection. The EWG (Environmental Working Group) introduced a new project called "Rethinking Cancer". It is a superb initiative offering educational blogs, research links, resources and an Ask the Expert section. They provide all this information for free, and only ask for donations to enable them to sustain their efforts. It is a group I gladly support!

 Would you find a basic **CLEAN PRODUCTS Cheat Sheet** *helpful? I have one for you to download right now. Click here if you are reading a digital book version*

http://www.kirstinscancercare.com/clean-products-cheat-sheet/

or find it at
www.kirstinscancercare.com/awesomebookbonuses/

CHAPTER 6
STEP 3
USE YOUR CONSCIOUS MIND

*"If we could get your subconscious mind to agree with your
conscious mind about being happy, that's when your
positive thoughts work."*
Bruce Lipton

Nothing really prepares you for the moment when you receive
the news that you have cancer yet again. I remember the very
first thoughts that raced through my mind were sheer, blunt
denial. "They must have confused the results. I have done so
much to heal, it can't be me!"

When reality hit hard and any doubt about dealing with the incor-
rect results had been gently removed by patient medical staff, a
sense of betrayal by my body and utter terror struck which, I will
admit, was not that easy to shake off at first.

"What else must I do?" "Did I not do enough?" "Do I really have
a fighting chance?" "Does everything I do really make a differ-

ence in the end?" Self-doubt and panic were the order of the day and it took a monumental effort to get myself grounded again and regain perspective on how I needed to approach my healing journey once again.

The most important part was allowing myself to release the emotions of fear, anger, guilt and despair. I could not think clearly beforehand. Thoughts and emotions are intertwined, dependent on each other, feeding off one another. While I was processing these very natural, but dark emotions, my mind was in what I refer to as 'Shadowland'. I knew I didn't belong there, and it was all surreal and undefined, no clear focused thought could emerge. I had no game plan, no clear way forward. It was important to surrender to this emotional release, which can scare the folks around you as it appears you are unraveling. The one who always had it together is teetering on the edge of hysteria.

I had another such moment when the news came from pathology after my bilateral mastectomy that the tissues and adjacent lymph nodes were riddled with cancerous cells at varying stages, none of which had been evident from all the diagnostic tests before surgery (besides thermography). It implied more extensive treatment than just the surgery. Again. Me, the one who actively embraced my first cancer completely holistically!

My quiet, introverted 14-year-old son said nothing when his 10-year old sister raced outside to the basketball hoop in our driveway to tell him this unexpected news, yet again. He simply dropped the ball, walked inside and proceeded to hug me, holding me tight for a very long time while I dissolved into a sobbing heap.

Such moments are part and parcel of a cancer journey, and are not at all a reflection of how strong or weak we are, or of how well we are coping, or not coping. We simply need to acknowledge that this intimate connection between thoughts and emotions, and likewise between emotions and thoughts, exists, is normal, and can be used to our advantage, or become a hindrance, when moving forward. We also need to understand that this interconnectedness can directly affect our physical body.

In my case, after emerging from Shadowland, and acknowledging that I did not get cancer again because I was to blame for not doing enough, or because I was doomed irrespective of what I did, my mind was sharp and focused again, back to the "me" that I knew could deal with anything because I have a will and determination to make the most of what this life wants me to achieve. I am here for a reason and purpose, and figuring that out, albeit challenging, is immensely rewarding.

This frame of mind was an essential step in nurturing myself back to health. I accepted the fact that there is more to learn in my life, and that despite my best efforts, there is never a guaranteed result. The exact outcome is not for me to decide. I am committed to addressing the root cause and to ultimately heal, whatever that may mean for me. And then I let go of just exactly how that healing is supposed to define itself for me.

Our thoughts, beliefs and emotions can have lasting impacts on the development of our disease as well as our overall healing capacity. The modern medical paradigm has made huge strides in eliminating infectious diseases and increasing our average lifespan through medical interventions, body part replacements and life-saving procedures.

It has systematically separated the mind from the body, and even though it recognizes certain aspects of the mind paradigm, such as the placebo effect, it still does not include a mind-healing regimen in mainstream recommendations or procedures. It just does not carry equal weight when it comes to devising a protocol to fight and heal from cancer.

Finding the right modality or mind technique is generally left to the individual. If you happen to mention this to your standard oncology team they may go as far as admitting that these are "good things" to include, and refer you to their lobby area where there may be schedules of different complementary modalities offered there. Having this on offer is a great improvement, and a huge step in the right direction.

Your traditional oncologist won't necessarily spend dedicated time educating you about the choices and options you have in this realm, and making sure that this is indeed a crucial element in your plan, because they have not been taught to do this. The current healthcare system in the US does not allow space, time or many resources, if any, for this. If certain cancer treatments are prescribed, wouldn't it be amazing if this would include mind-body techniques as an indispensable, and health-insurance-covered, part of your regimen? It would send out such a strong signal of the importance of a mind-body approach when dealing with chronic diseases such as cancer.

One of the first books I devoured was Deb Shapiro's "*Your Body Speaks Your Mind – Understanding How Your Emotions and Thoughts Affect You Physically*", As she aptly states, an overlooked part of one's healing process is an understanding that "the mind and body are not two but one single body mind" in which "every part of the body is the mind expressing itself through that part". We need to get in touch with our bodies to understand the "intimate two-way communication" that affects our physical body as well as our mental and emotional health.

How can the mind be so powerful as to elicit a physical reaction? With all due respect to the complex dynamics making up our body, allow me to reduce it here to this: our thoughts and feelings are directly connected to our nervous system, both central and autonomous, our mother ship. Our nervous system steers numerous bodily functions such as the immune system, endocrine system, digestive system, respiratory system and blood circulation by way of chemical messengers such as our hormones, neurotransmitters and neuropeptides that are continuously being sent all over the body even during our sleep. (Shapiro).

Every thought, and every associated emotion, triggers the release of such chemical messengers that elicit a physical consequence, either a health-supporting, or a balance-disrupting one.

You are familiar with the saying: You are what you eat! Let's add to that: You are what you think! One is not more important than the other. They are equally important. What you eat is your choice! What you think is your choice too!

Just as the food you put in your mouth can serve as pure nourishment, a pharmacy or a toxic dump, so can your mind become instrumental in contributing to how you, as a living organism, can deal with what you are exposed to.

Being alive means being subjected to stressful situations; it is part of our normal existence and it has ensured our long-term survival. Knowing how to respond to a life-threatening situation has ensured we could get ourselves out of dangerous situations, and this reaction was as a result of the mechanisms we have in place to deal with stress.

We are programmed to respond. How we respond is something we program ourselves. That is our choice. We may be conditioned to respond in a certain way, due to perhaps what we have become accustomed to, or how we have seen others react. Often it is a habitual pattern we may fall into without consciously realizing that we are doing it.

One of my clients, with advanced stage rectal cancer knew very well that she was consciously contributing to a major stress factor in her life by allowing her verbally abusive adult son to continue to live with her. She even admitted to having lost friends along the way who were exasperated by this intolerable situation. Her response to my question why she was knowingly allowing this major stress to be a part of her life, was simply this: "I have always done it this way, and know I should do something about it, but it's too late now."

Interestingly, when you consider that she had cancer in the rectum, this is the final point of elimination from the body, connected to the mouth as the first entry point. The rectum is a private part that, energetically, can store feelings of abuse and violation. As Shapiro explains the body-mind dialogue in the case of the rectum concerns the question "is someone being a pain in the backside" and "are they getting too close and invading my privacy?" By deciding not to do anything about her son's relentless verbal abuse of her, even though she knew she should have done so years ago, energetically she was holding on to all that tension and stored feelings in her rectum. Unfortunately, it was too late for her to let go and find out.

It is ultimately within our power to decide with which attitude we confront our lives. And to change if we realize the path we are on is not serving us anymore. Do we wish to remain a victim of circumstance, or do we see a much higher purpose for our life? We can choose differently.

Cancer is a red flag waved right under our nose that alerts us to the fact that the way we have lived our life up to that point, may not be health-supporting. In particular, we need to take a closer look at how we respond to the stress factors in our lives.

I want to illustrate this by an example of what I consider a major stressful situation. Although I knew what type of details this autobiography might entail, I was drawn to read the story of Immaculaeé Illibagiza, author of *"Left to Tell"* and survivor of the Rwandan genocide in the 1990's. After reading it in almost one sitting, I knew what attracted me to it so much.

It is a hugely inspiring tale of sheer will and intention to survive, not only the physical life threatening danger Immaculaeé was subjected to, but also the mental trauma that resulted in the aftermath of the horrific tragedy that vividly displayed what can happen when friends and neighbors turn against each other in a frenzy of gruesome accusations and brutal killings.

During the 1994 Rwandan genocide Immaculaeé hid in a tiny bathroom for three months together with a group of six other women in a space so confined they had to partly lie on top of each other, to escape, and hopefully remain undetected from the mobs of killers that were raiding the areas. They were hidden by a soul of a man who risked his and his family's lives, secretly feeding them sporadically from left-overs, so that not even his family noticed. Immaculaeé survived, but her entire family, except for one brother, were brutally murdered.

This trauma could be a fertile internal environment for cancer cells to have a field day. However, Immaculaeé rose above this and is an inspirational and motivational speaker today. How did she achieve this?

She consciously chose her Catholic faith to help her through the actual stressful time as it was happening to her. She used the power of her mind to keep her wits about her when she was physically unable to do anything but be a sitting duck for a possible gruesome end to her life. She had no control over what would happen to her, but she could control her mind. She spent most of the three months in prayer, trying to get her mind off the fear, hunger, dehydration and extreme physical discomfort.

After she was rescued, she instinctively knew that she had to adopt an additional mental healing tool for the trauma she witnessed not to destroy her ultimately. She chose to allow space for forgiveness despite the deep emotional pain and raw anger she was feeling. With the help of her faith, she chose to find out the details of what happened to her family members, and then sought out to locate the murderers that were still alive and imprisoned by then, most of whom she knew, to personally forgive them. A heroic action in my opinion!

She used the power of her thoughts, beliefs and emotions to overcome the psychological trauma that very well could have overshadowed the life she was spared. She could have been stuck in the trauma of her experiences for the rest of her life, and chances would have been high that this trauma could result in the manifestation of a physical disease.

In my personal healing quest to understand just how powerful a tool this concept of the mind being able to influence the outcome of what happens within my body can be, I came across this fascinating study.

Dr. Masaru Emoto, a Japanese scientist, started out experimenting with water crystals to explore the concept that no single water crystal is alike. He was hoping to obtain information about the state of water. He began photographing frozen water with a high-resolution microscope, and discovered that there was a difference in the physical appearance of water depending on where he had sourced it.

Natural spring water had a very different structure when frozen than water collected from a kitchen tap. The shape of the crystal was either beautifully formed, or incomplete.

He deducted from this that something gave the water molecules the information to either be stable and thus able to form a complete crystal when frozen, or not. So he became motivated to explore what would happen if you began to influence this information in different ways.

Rather than being a passive observer, he actively started to influence the state of water by subjecting it to different immediate environments. He and his team started playing music to water while still in its liquid state, and were astounded to see how the shape of the crystal was directly influenced by what music the water was subjected to.

They discovered that water reacted to sound vibrations and was able to store this information in its own way, to be used when having to form a crystal when it was subjected to freezing temps. Classical music, Gregorian chants, Buddhist mantras and contemporary pop music was used and produced profoundly different results.

They went one step further. In Japanese culture they believe that every word has a soul, and carries with it specific vibrations related to an emotion associated with the word. They labeled different water bottles with different words, and you can probably guess what I am about to reveal.

Water labeled with the word demon produced distorted and discolored crystals, whereas words like love, gratitude, peace produced perfectly-shaped, brightly-colored ones. It was as if the meaning of the word influenced the actual shape. A whole phrase like "giving birth" showed a crystal with dynamic, developing movement. "The healing hands of the mother" produced a slight pink color, a color which is associated with activating life energy.

So, what is our take-away from this story? Words create vibrations that can alter the structural state of water, and these vibrations can be stored. Considering we are made up of about 70% water, this is quite a stunning theory.

When we are thinking a thought, we give it energy by saying it out aloud or imagining it as real. This pattern of vibration is stored within us, and we reflect it outward too, thus influencing the environment around us. Others react to this, and give us the appropriate feedback that can reinforce our vibrations, and so the cycle of creation can keep us in a state of being that may or may not be beneficial to us at that time.

I know what you may be thinking now (no pun intended). Thinking different thoughts sounds like a simple thing to do, but how do we do it? How do we influence habitual thinking patterns that keep us enslaved, despite our attempts to redirect them? Can we really influence our physical reality, just by thinking different thoughts?

I, like you, wondered whether I could train myself to think more positively and whether this would have a direct, measurable outcome in my life? Should I begin to write down a list of positive affirmations that I read to myself on a daily basis? I discovered that while there is most certainly some benefit to this practice, we have to take it a step further.

I credit my "A-HA moment" to discovering the fascinating principles of Quantum Physics, and in particular to two influential and inspiring researchers and educators in the field of neuro-science, Dr. Bruce Lipton and Dr. Joe Dispenza.

In their groundbreaking books *"The Biology of Belief: Unleashing the Power of Consciousness, Matter and Miracles"* by Dr. Bruce Lipton and *"Breaking the Habit of Being Yourself – How to Lose Your Mind and Create an New One" by* Dr. Joe Dispenza, they each illustrate through their research how you can reprogram your thinking through scientifically proven neuro-physiological principles, based on quantum physics.

In order to understand where they are coming from, let's digress a little to provide a brief background about Mind over Matter theory and how it has evolved over the last hundreds of years from one which stated that mind and matter were always separate, and that one could not influence the other, to the quantum physics-based notion that both are one and the same.

The 17th Century mathematician Descartes, the originator of the "I think therefore I am" philosophy, made striding contributions to our understanding of mathematics and science even to this day, but in one aspect he started a belief system that split mind and matter into separate and mutually exclusive camps.

He stated that the Universe is controlled by predictable laws and matter was always to be explained by scientific study. Mind, however, fell under the jurisdiction of God, this was the realm of religion and always separate from matter.

Sir Isaac Newton perpetuated this belief system and came up with a set of laws that enabled humans to operate the physical world by precise calculations and predictions. All things were considered solid, and energy can be explained as simply an outside force that moves objects or changes the physical state of things. Reality was mechanistic, and humans could not actually control the outcomes. Humans are purely on the receiving end of any action.

In 1900 German Physicist Max Planck proved that energy is not just a wave-like phenomenon, but is made up of little particles, each called a "quantum". Energy can effectively display characteristics of physical matter. Then Albert Einstein appeared with his radical new scientific revelation that energy and matter are so fundamentally related that they are actually one and the same. Both are completely interchangeable. This was a direct contradiction to the rigid thinking of the Descartes and Newtonian principles.

Einstein's theory sparked widespread research into the principles of light. Light sometimes behaved like a wave (energy), when it bends around a corner, and sometimes like a particle (matter). How could that be? If they could be either or both, what was it then? What could you reduce this to? What is the tiniest component of everything? Scientists of the day scrambled to uncover the mysteries of this revolutionary new concept. A new field of science was born - quantum physics.

This is not a Science 101 lesson, but I am telling you this so that you can see how scientifically-based this perhaps esoteric notion of thoughts being able to change the physical nature of things, actually is.

Quantum physics changed an understanding of a world we thought we had figured out. We had been taught (Newtonian principle) that the tiniest component is an atom, a solid piece of structure with a definite nucleus and electrons swirling around it in measured oval-shaped patterns.

Not so. A Quantum Atom is considered to be mostly energy, with a nucleus and the probability of the space around it being taken up by an electron. Think about the implication thereof. Everything physical in our lives is not necessarily solid matter, but fields of energy, or frequency patterns of information.

So, what makes this book a solid structure then? What makes it real?

According to Quantum Physics, our mindful attention! The energy in everything responds to mindful attention and then shapes into a form that we can see and feel like a physical structure.

Quantum Physicists discovered that the person observing the tiny particles that make up atoms directly affect the behavior of energy and matter. The electrons exist simultaneously in an infinite array of possibilities in an invisible field of energy. Only when an observer focuses the attention on any one location, does an electron appear.

A particle does not become real unless we observe it – the classic "observer effect". This showed irrevocably that the subjective mind can produce a change in the physical world that is fully measurable.

What does that mean for us? The energy that is the basis of us, that is most of us, responds to our mindful attention and can become matter.

As Dr. Joe Dispenza puts it this way: "You are powerful enough to influence matter because at the most elementary level, you are energy with consciousness. You are a mindful matter".

All possibilities for reality exist in the quantum field around us, just waiting for a conscious observer to come along and turn these energy waves into physical matter. We are more than just a physical body (matter). We are a consciousness using a body and a brain to express different levels of mind.

We communicate with the quantum field through our thoughts and emotions. These thoughts are energy, and these electrical impulses can be measured by devices like an EEG (electroen-cephalogram).

The HeartMath Research Center in California has dedicated 24 years of scientific research into the study of the physiology of emotions, learning and performance. In 2003 they conducted a study to see whether human intention could change the structure of DNA. They showed that negative emotions produce erratic and disorganized heart rhythms, while positive thoughts elicit highly ordered, coherent patterns. Based on this premise they conducted this fascinating study.

Three groups of participants, each holding vials with DNA samples, were involved. The first group held the vials while producing strong positive feelings of love and appreciation. No significant changes were found in the DNA.

The second group produced the same strong positive feelings and held an intention, a specific thought, to either wind or unwind the strands of DNA. Significant changes in the shape of the DNA were noted, up to a 25% change in some.

The third group held the clear intention to wind or unwind the DNA, but no simultaneous positive emotions. No changes to the DNA samples were recorded.

Only when participants used both thoughts and emotions did a change in the DNA structure of the genes in the vials occur. When only one or the other was used, the desired effect wasn't achieved.

What does that imply? A thought, an intention, needs to be paired with a strong emotion to create a state of being. The quantum field does not simply respond to our wishes, or just our thoughts, both have to be combined to produce the desired effect.

As Dr. Dispenza puts it, "the Quantum field responds not to what we want, but to who we are being". If we send out the same thoughts and feelings, we create the same behaviors and thus the same reality.

If we want to change our reality, we need to **become someone else**. When we send out this new being into the field, it will meet its equivalent potential in the field and we will be pulled toward that potential reality, or it will find us.

One important thing to consider in this theory: we should not try to control the outcome of our intention, as then we are back to the Newtonian way of wanting to predict events and create a cause and effect, allowing the outside environment to control our thinking.

The quantum view is the other way around: change your internal environment – the way you think and feel – and then sit back and observe how the outside environment responds. Just think and feel the "what", leave the "how" up to the field. It's challenging us to change our thoughts and feelings before the event has materialized. We should feel as if the reality has already happened.

When I was first diagnosed, I was in the middle of furthering my education and was back at school, studying. My mid-term exams were around the corner when I was diagnosed and having to undergo surgery and start treatments. My lecturers were all very supportive and the Institute offered to postpone my exams; they told me I could write them whenever I had recovered and felt up to it.

It was all you could ask for, and I was very grateful for their understanding and willingness to accommodate me. However, that is not what I needed right then. My diagnosis spurred me on to become an expert in exactly that niche – supporting people with cancer, people like me.

I wanted that focus. I wanted to write that exam with everyone else. I did not want to be exempt. I needed it now more than ever, so I decided that I was going to do this and study while I was recovering from my surgery. It was the best medicine I could have asked for right then.

It was having a purpose, and seeing myself successfully helping others, that helped me harness an empowering attitude to get me through those first few months of diagnosis and treatment. I had a long-term goal I wanted to accomplish, and cancer was not going to throw me off this path. I was not just going to survive this, but go on to what I actually wanted to do, even if the pace and direction might be a little different than I envisioned before my diagnosis.

Although I initially viewed my cancer as a stumbling block I had to figure out how best to navigate around it; it soon became my jump board that catapulted me into a world of personal discovery and self-growth I could not possibly have attained without my diagnosis.

And then my world turned upside down again when I was diagnosed a second time, three short years later. I had just started my own nutrition consulting practice. I was full of optimistic enthusiasm and ready to help anyone who wanted to learn how to lead a healthier life. Receiving the diagnosis was as though I was stopped in my tracks. Why on earth was I not supposed to do what I thought was my path?

From a conscious mind point of view, my second breast cancer was a lesson in ultimate acceptance and surrender towards life and my role within it. It is not up to me to decide where my path is heading, only to know that I have a path to travel, with various stops along the way that I consider life lessons in compassion and humility, first and foremost to ourselves.

I do not mean by this that we simply sit back and wait for life to unfold. Far from it. We are fully responsible for our choice of paths, and need to actively engage in moving forward, backward or sideways. We have a goal and we project ourselves into that vision, and then we release how we are going to get there and simply focus our consciousness on this moment in time. In this moment we accept responsibility for our choices; we accept or reject opportunities that present themselves and we understand that nothing is 100% perfect or guaranteed.

We incorporate a more conscious approach to what really matters in our lives. We become aware of exactly what we are thinking during a day, a week, a month. And we choose to redirect any negative thoughts or reactionary behaviors that no longer serve us.

At a time of my life when I was stuck on just how I was supposed to do this, a colleague gave me a book entitled, *"A Complaint Free*

World – How to Stop Complaining and Start Enjoying the Life You Always Wanted" by Will Bowen. It contains a 21-Day Challenge to help you develop a different habit that lasts. He started this in his congregation, and by now millions of people have taken him up on it.

It is very simple and costs you absolutely nothing, but pure mindfulness. Using a bracelet or wristband of choice, every time you find yourself thinking a negative thought, such as complaining, criticizing or gossiping either verbally or in your head over the next 21 days, move the bracelet to the other wrist.

You will be amazed at how many times you will be doing this in the beginning. You will slowly see how the frequency changes, and you become more aware of your thoughts so that you will be able to stop yourself from even thinking in that direction. That is what you want to achieve. Conscious mindfulness to break an old habit and internalize a new one. Go ahead and try it. I challenge you to do this starting right now! It is a life-changing little exercise to get you accustomed to thinking different thoughts, changing your words, and finding a different path in your life.

Another exercise you can try is starting a daily gratitude journal, but a little differently than you may have done before. To gain perspective and appreciate what we actually have, it is a common practice to list things we are grateful for that are already in our lives.

I have found this a very useful exercise to become grounded again and realize all the positive influences and achievements that are already an integral part of my life. There is nothing fundamentally wrong with this at all. But in the quantum view, let's give thanks for something we don't have yet, *as if* we already have it.

If this sounds radical to you now, allow yourself to digest it for a little bit. I know this concept is a giant leap of faith! It certainly was for me, and sometimes still is as I slowly begin to adjust to this concept and unravel years of imprinted thinking in my brain.

If this subject interests you, Dr. Dispenza offers a step-by-step meditation CD to accompany his book *"Breaking the Habit of Being Yourself"*. I found it riveting; it helped me get into the state of mind that makes so much sense to me. And as a bonus, I got my husband on board too, the ever-skeptical engineer. He appreciated the scientific background to the theory.

It is not my intention to "convert" you to this way of thinking, I simply wish to share what I have come across when I was searching for answers, as I knew that "positive thinking" on its own was simply not enough to really set things in motion. What you choose to believe in is essentially your business, please see this simply as a collection of information I have found viable, evidence-based and worthy of presenting to you.

 Would you like a quick head start? Click here to download my **3 STEPS TO RETRAIN YOUR BRAIN Worksheet** *right now if you are reading a digital book version*

http://www.kirstinscancercare.com/3-steps-retrain-brain-worksheet/

or find it at
www.kirstinscancercare.com/awesomebookbonuses/

Chapter 7

STEP 4
Allow emotional healing

"Trying to suppress or eradicate symptoms on the physical level can be extremely important, but there's more to healing than that; dealing with psychological, emotional and spiritual issues involved in treating sickness is equally important."
Marianne Williamson

When my now teenage daughter was one year old a friend and I attended a two-day workshop by the Omega Institute in New York. It was my first immersion into the infinite possibilities of a Mind-Body approach to health and healing.

One workshop I chose to attend became the trigger for my own personal journey of growth and transformation, and, years later, would be the spark that led me to unravel the root cause of my cancers, although I did not know the impact it would have on me at the time.

It was a workshop held by Dr. Brian Weiss, MD, chairman emeritus of psychiatry at the Mount Sinai Medical Center in Miami and a leading authority in the US on past-life regression therapy. I had no clue what this was going to be about, but found the subject intriguing.

To illustrate his presentation he offered a group hypnosis session, and seeing that I was in a room of over 250 people all I needed to do was close my eyes, and allow myself to become deeply relaxed through a guided visualization he spoke us through.

This experience changed my life, although not immediately as the effects of it had to sink in and percolate through my conditioned way of thinking and how linearly I had approached life up until that point.

During the group session I became so deeply relaxed that I could see myself moving toward a door surrounded by bright light, but I could not go through it, it stayed shut and I had no idea how to go forward.

Tears started flowing, but I was not crying. It was unlike any other tearful release I had ever experienced before. Somehow I knew I needed to get through that door, but it wasn't the right time yet. I also knew it wasn't symbolic of my death. All the while I was still present in my chair in that room full of people, I could hear what was going on around me but it was all at a distance and I was comfortable being so relaxed.

When Dr. Weiss guided us into full consciousness again and I opened my eyes, I felt incredibly at peace, but there was a yearning in me as I knew that I needed to explore this realm more. Why and exactly how I did not know at the time. I recall being impressed that hypnosis did not mean I drifted off into Neverland, not knowing what people could have me do for other people's amusement, which is the general association most people have when they hear "hypnosis". This hypnotherapy technique was nothing more than deep relaxation at free will, remaining fully conscious the entire time, remembering every-thing that went on around me.

Fast forward about six years, when I was diagnosed with my first breast cancer, when that inner yearning stirred up again and despite being consumed by the raw shock of the news, I instinc-tively knew the time had come to explore this further and enter through that brightly lit door. I knew it would open up for me now, and that this would lead me to answers I was desperately seeking, way beyond the typical explanation of "it's my turn now", which was the obvious and logical assumption consider-ing my family history.

After my Omega Institute workshop, I read one of Dr. Weiss' books *"Through Time into Healing – Discovering the Power of Regression Therapy to Erase Trauma and Transform Mind, Body and Relationships"*. Dr. Weiss, a traditional psychotherapist, stum-bled across hypnosis-based regression therapy by chance as he was trying to help a client of his suffering from severe fears, phobias and panic attacks that were not improving even though she had been seeing him for quite some time.

Agreeing to use hypnosis as a focused attention session, the client was able to access information stored in her subconscious mind that explained why she was experiencing her present-day physical and mental symptoms. In trying to get to the root cause of her symptoms, she not only recalled events from her early childhood, but from past lives as well, in which she experienced certain traumatic events that mirrored her current present day issues. After these sessions, she slowly began to improve and her symptoms disappeared as she understood how this trapped trauma had still been influencing her to this day, releasing it in the process.

At this personal turning point in my life, I recalled Dr. Weiss' case studies and how they had fascinated me a few years back. My inquisitive nature surfaced again, the incessant "why?" questions that are simply not satisfied with the conventional reasons offered as the usual answers for why I probably got cancer.

In his book *"Heal Thyself"*, Dr. Pieter De Wet, MD, an integrative doctor, who has dedicated his medical career to helping redress root causes and allow true healing for thousands of patients over the past 30 years, gives a candid view of why we end up getting sick. Each manifested disease, cancer included, is a reflection of an internal conflict that started out on a psychological level. If allowed to increase in intensity, it begins to overwhelm the brain, which tries to balance this stress with normal bodily functions. This overwhelm causes the unresolved conflict to become physiological, resulting in physical symptoms in certain body parts that, according to Dr. De Wet, "correspond to the exact tonality of the conflict".

In his view, an initial "programming conflict", as he refers to it, on its own may not necessarily lead to an illness, however it can pave the way in the brain and corresponding body organ or tissue for the potential disease to take root in the future. A "triggering conflict" in the form of another, often unrelated, event can then kick-start this dormant conflict, compounding the stress, and an illness can manifest. Sometimes the programming conflict occurred years before, and was not even necessarily a typical traumatic event such as the death of a loved one or a major accident.

It can be an experience from childhood when we were overlooked or punished perhaps for something we did not commit. This experience left an emotional imprint which, if exposed to a triggering conflict years later, can exacerbate the stress response, leading to an overreaction and an outbreak of, for example, cancer. Dr. De Wet also points to the fact that often such an outbreak can happen after we have resolved an issue in our lives and the body is in a healing release state, yet the pre-existing biological pathways have been set in motion and will run their course.

This may explain why sometimes we are diagnosed with cancer even though our lives seem to run smoothly, and we cannot associate a particular incident with getting cancer at that point. Or we lead what we consider to be pretty healthy lifestyles already, yet we get diagnosed and cannot figure out why we, as a healthy person, are not spared.

I see this more frequently with clients who are eating an already impressive diet, are fit, exercise regularly and practice some form of self-care, yet still get diagnosed and are flummoxed why it hit them. Invariably, none of them have dealt with any deep-rooted emotional component to their lives, although they can point out issues where they think there could be a possible association.

I knew what my emotional association was right away too, and did not hesitate to call on a dear friend and professional hypnotherapist to help me uncover what I clearly was not accessing with my conscious mind. My mother and I had a very troubled and challenging relationship once I became an adolescent, and up to that point had not been able to resolve this underlying, simmering disconnect that seemed to flare up every so often.

Whenever we had an incident I would feel real physical pain in my upper torso, an area akin to the heart chakra energy center. It felt like I was on fire there. So I knew there was something I needed to do about it, just that I did not know where to start, and kept ignoring this warning sign clearly sent to alert me to a psycho-physical imbalance that needed my attention.

Not only was this a "programming conflict", as Dr. De Wet would call it, but also a "triggering conflict" as this was a situation that affected me for years, each time leaving an energetic imprint I ignored, and growing in magnitude as little incidents over the years kept on adding to the issue.

My subsequent hypnotherapy sessions were mind-blowing, excuse the pun, as the boundaries of my conscious mind were explosively expanded as I gained an insight into what was going on at a subconscious level. I got a glimpse of who I really am, what I am capable of, if I allow it, and how emotional imprints of past experiences can keep us enslaved until we consciously decide to release them.

The resulting feeling of utter liberation, boundlessness and crystal clarity was so tangible it was physically noticeable. I will never forget my husband's expression when he saw me after my first hypnotherapy session, which was pretty intense as I was ready to go through that door this time, and flinging open wide for me it certainly did! "Your eyes are completely changed, what the heck happened to you?" Apparently I radiated peace and he could actually feel it in the house. My energy field had shifted, and people around me noticed.

In the previous chapter I referred to how our thoughts carry energetic vibrations that can influence how we recover and heal from cancer. We can impact this by making a conscious decision to redirect any negative thoughts and change reactionary behaviors that are not conducive to healing.

When we want to address suppressed emotions, we need to move beyond our conscious thoughts and allow access to the many layers of our subconscious minds. If this sounds somewhat frightening to you, and you may even ask: "Why would I want to subject myself to possibly re-living this trauma again?" then allow me to put your mind at ease.

Ensuring a free flow of life energy is a very common modality in eastern health traditions, and we see its many uses in our western society today. Yoga, gi qong, tai chi, acupuncture or acupressure are just a few examples that have made it to mainstream practice today. Even chiropractic adjustments can lead to the release of certain emotional connections to physical imbalances, often referred to as subluxations. All of these methods have one central theme: allowing the body to self-regulate and enable it to remove any blockages to the free flow of our life energy, and thus the capacity to heal fully.

Suppressed emotional trauma can be seen as such blockages. They can be present at a conscious level (we can remember and recall them) or at a subconscious level (we cannot consciously remember or recall anything). Certain traumatic experiences are deliberately blocked from one's memories, but the energetic vibrations are still there, and in essence, block our immune systems from being able to function optimally.

Dr. Bradley Nelson, MD, in his Book *"The Emotion Code – How to Release Your Trapped Emotions for Abundant Health, Love and Happiness,"* reiterates how "trapped emotions are truly epidemic, and are the insidious, invisible cause of much suffering and illness, both physical and emotional in nature."

He likens having a trapped emotion a bit like having a tuning fork in your body that will proceed to vibrate at the same frequency of that negative emotion, affecting its surrounding environment and even attracting more of the same emotion, causing a vicious circle of negative emotional resonance.

How we access and release them is a very personal choice, and I will outline a few other options below besides hypnotherapy. We choose what resonates with us, and we may even move from one modality to another as we progress on our healing journey.

Based on having experienced this myself and having seen my clients shift their relationships with cancer, recognizing that to address all the root causes we have to include an emotional healing component is, in my opinion, not optional. It is an integral part of our healing regimen.

If you are still unsure of committing to this step, ask yourself what exactly you are afraid of. I mean this in the most non-judgmental way possible as we are all faced with this at some point or another, myself included. Fear of the unknown, of "what may come up" can be a major stumbling block for some of us. However, you do not need to go along this path alone!

Whatever emotional healing modality you choose to start with, I highly recommend finding a professional energy healing practitioner to guide you through this healing process. Although certain self-help tools can, and should be used along the way, to address the deeper layers of consciousness we need to entrust ourselves to someone who knows how to steer us through the process of emotional release. This way, we are not re-experiencing this trauma as in real life, but as a passing observer with a secured exit and warmth and healing energy at the end point. It cannot threaten us anymore, but rather liberate us from the bonds in which it kept us for so long, even if we did not realize this.

I started out with hypnotherapy sessions because I had encountered the process before, and I knew the person whom I entrusted this soul ride to. I still use this modality now and then, but I have also branched out and explored others as I continuously stay on this path of self-discovery and self-healing, seeing my layers unfold and my consciousness reaching deeper levels within.

It has helped me understand the dynamics in my life as they unfold, the relationships I have with my immediate family, close friends, clients, acquaintances and even strangers I may meet only once. We are all interconnected somehow, and our individual and combined energies bounce around, off each other, sometimes in a rhythmic dance and sometimes in a combustive explosion.

When I was diagnosed a second time, I knew intuitively that it was not a recurrence, but a different cancer, even though that had not been determined diagnostically yet. How could I be so sure?

Before my first diagnosis, and over the course of many years, I had consciously worked on coming to terms with the relationship I had with my mother at the time, or so I thought. As mentioned earlier, the fact that I, at times, experienced real heart pain after interacting with her should have told me that I had not dealt with the emotional baggage attached to this at all. Physical symptoms like this are always a warning signal, without fail. Only once I delved into the subconscious mind and allowed that to bubble up did I truly release these emotional ties.

How do I know I received the "all clear"? The best way is always direct confrontation and waiting for the tell-tale signs of tension to present themselves. Now to explain a little, my mother and I did not have any arguments or heated word exchanges over the past years anymore, we both had avoided this and circumnavigated sensitive issues where we knew we were of very different opinions. The effects were a lot more subtle; sometimes just being energetically connected on the phone would set off this heart pain within me.

I knew I was in for the challenge when my parents decided to visit us in the US for the first time in nine years, spending three weeks with us which they had never before done since I moved out of their house seventeen years previously.

Would my buttons be pushed? I admit I was a little nervous, as I truly believed I had released it all, and wanted this success to be validated. I could not have hoped for a more perfect verification of the power of emotional release at a subconscious level.

Throughout her stay, all I felt was pure love. I saw her for the struggling soul she was, as we all are at times, connected on the same plane, even though she was still my mother in all aspects. Interestingly, I saw a part of her behavior having the same effect on my then eight-year-old daughter as it had on me all those years ago, and luckily could help my little confused girl by applying some energetic release work that could help diffuse the underlying tension.

Needless to say, I was thrilled to be completely free of any heart pain or resentment, and could just enjoy the presence of my mother and give her the love that I am sure she had yearned for from me all those years. I intuitively felt it was the last time I would see her, and I was at peace with this. She passed away very suddenly only five days after returning home, and although this was an unexpected shock, I had expected it to happen very soon.

I am mentioning this personal story to illustrate how important it is to heed the signs and work on "our stuff" while we still have the ability to test that our work is complete.

Looking back, it was important for me to go through it all while she was still alive. I feel very blessed that I was able to send just the pure love she deserved to feel from me because I had done the subconscious work of releasing the emotional trauma between us, spanning many life times, that had soured most of our adult relationship. It could not have been resolved through conscious interaction between us during our time together as this trauma sat deep in my subconscious realm. I also accepted that she would have to deal with her issues on her own, and that I was not responsible for this. She was still the same she had always been. The shift had been in me, and she noticed this too as it positively affected how I reacted to her during her visit.

That's the reason why I could intuitively feel that the under-lying emotional cause of my first cancer was dealt with. Please understand, knowing this does not make it any easier to accept a second diagnosis! When the pathology report showed different cancer markers, I was once again thrown onto the next roller-coaster wagon of "what the heck is it now?"

It wasn't as obvious to me as it was on my first round, and this is important to mention. This time around I did not know immedi-ately which relationship or area in my life I needed to focus on to clear any suppressed emotional baggage.

It took some time to figure out that I needed to adopt a more conscious approach that had personal self-esteem, feelings of worthiness and life purpose issues at heart. We can self-sabo-tage ourselves both at a conscious and subconscious level. This process of unearthing these underlying emotional dynamics requires a very frank and personal date with yourself and all your quirks and habits. It is one of the hardest things to do as we always focus on everyone else, but ourselves.

Here are some different **energy healing modalities** I have used personally over the years with great success. Please note there are numerous methods you can choose from, I have limited my list here to those I have experienced myself, and still regularly use when the need arises.

I want to present you with a basic overview only, as my inten-tion is not to teach you about these modalities, but to showcase just some of the many options you can choose from in order to achieve a very similar result: addressing and releasing any sup-pressed emotional blockages you may have so that healing can take place at this level as well. If after reading these summaries you feel drawn to a specific technique, I have given you further reading and websites for you to explore.

Neuro Emotional Technique (NET)

Neuro Emotional Technique is a neuro-emotional stress reduction intervention aimed at physical as well as emotional health improvement. It is very effective at finding the origins of emotional trauma, with the help of muscle testing and applying pressure to acupressure points along the meridian-energy system.

This principle that links emotions with energy meridians, or invisible pathways along the body, has a traditional medicine history dating back thousands of years, and is key in the Traditional Chinese Medicine Approach. The recipient is muscle tested by a practitioner, but applies the acupressure on certain points mainly on the wrists and head themselves during a session.

A session typically starts off with a question and answer discussion where the therapist will try to pinpoint an area of concern that you wish to focus on. Sometimes, this alone can take you to a place where you have a "bingo" moment and may tear up or become agitated as certain associated emotions come up for you. At this point the therapy will shift to you becoming the instigator and releasing this emotional pain with the NET method. It is a truly interactive session, and empowering as you, the patient, actively release anything that needs to be cleared, right in one session.

A study published in the *Journal of Cancer Survivorship* in 2007 showed that stress symptoms related to traumatic cancer-events in a group of women survivors, who did not qualify as meeting the criteria for post-traumatic stress disorder (PTSD), were relieved with the intervention of NET.

In a more recent study published in the same journal in 2017, which intended to test whether the NET-induced processing of traumatic memories associated with a cancer-related event could be observed showing up as physiological changes in the brain, a marked reduction in emotional stress was observed in the patients tested. Once again, it is encouraging to see such positive measurable results with the use of a mind-body technique to help people heal from cancer.

> **Recommended Website:**
> https://www.netmindbody.com/for-patients/an-explanation-of-net

Eye Movement Desensitization and Reprocessing (EMDR)

EMDR is a recognized psychotherapy tool, initiated by psychologist Dr. Francine Shapiro in the late 1980's, when she was treating Vietnam veterans for PTSD (post-traumatic stress disorder). EMDR allows people who have undergone traumatic or negative experiences to heal from the emotional distress these have caused.

EMDR therapy offers a relatively quick way for the mind to release stored emotional trauma. By voluntarily using rapid eye movements, similarly to what we encounter involuntarily during REM sleep, and associating them with certain negative memories of past events, a recipient can begin processing these memories on an emotional level.

By being guided by a psychotherapist at a particular point of recall during a session to rapidly move the eyes from left to right, both sides of the brain are stimulated, activating the nervous system to release stuck experiences.

The recipient takes full ownership as the release happens upon own stimulation, not at the suggestion of a therapist. This is a very empowering process as the recipient steers the progress and can actively let go of negative emotional associations that can arise during a session.

It is quite fascinating to experience this as you sit still, across from the therapist, and follow a pointer with your eyes from left to right, and back again, at a particular pace. At that point you have recalled a situation that has caused you distress, based on the discussion you had previously with your therapist. What happens is that an associated emotion, or a connection to a past event, pops up in your mind out of nowhere, or so it seems. It actually is being released by your mind during this stimulation, and that release alone can be enough to clear that issue from your subconscious as well as conscious mind.

It is promising to see that in the past five years an increasing number of studies on the effectiveness of EMDR are being conducted. One such study published in the journal *Psychological Trauma* in 2016 concluded that active duty service members with PTSD (post-traumatic stress disorder) receiving EMDR needed far fewer therapy sessions than those undergoing traditional therapy. Other studies are exploring the use of EMDR in patients suffering from chronic pain. Further randomized control studies are still needed, but the initial findings are very encouraging.

> **Recommended Website:** http://www.emdr.com/
>
> **Recommended reading:** *"Getting Past your Past: Take Control of Your Life with Self-Help Techniques from EMDR Therapy"* by Francine Shapiro

Reiki

Receiving a Reiki session is a calming, relaxing experience where universal healing energy is being channeled through the attuned practitioner into the recipient by laying on hands in a hovering position, not necessarily via direct touch.

It is based on the premise that our life force energy is affected by thoughts and emotions, and can become disrupted if we accept negative thoughts about ourselves. Universal healing energy, channeled through the Reiki practitioner, raises vibrational frequencies of affected body parts. In essence, it is not the practitioner that creates the healing experience, he or she just enables the process to happen naturally. Anyone can benefit from this non-invasive healing modality.

I am an attuned Reiki practitioner myself and have applied Reiki to clients, my family, our dogs and myself. It is an amazing experience when you place your hands above certain areas of the body, guided by the intuitive direction of where to hover for a while, and then receive a tingling, hot sensation as a confirmation that energy is being channeled. It is a very relaxing, and passive experience for the receiver.

I remember during my first round of chemo, before I was attuned myself, I had fallen off my bike onto my right knee, and was in agony. That day I visited a close friend who happened to be a

Reiki practitioner. She saw me hobble through her door, told me to sit down and while we chatted away just held her hand over it. Intense, but soothing heat radiated through my knee and leg for the entire time. When I left for home I walked solidly on that leg with the pain having subsided by about 80%. I was amazed! I decided to become a practitioner myself, as this is also a valuable self-help tool that you can apply anywhere, anytime.

Recommended website:
http://www.reiki.org/

Spiritual Response Therapy (SRT)

SRT is another way of finding out which energetic or spiritual blockages could be the underlying causes for problems or issues in a person's life. This technique is based on the notion that the subconscious mind can give a signal or clue, also referred to as an ideomotor response that can shed light on what is going on under the surface of the conscious mind. A thought or an emotion can cause a physical reaction in the body, such as a tiny muscular twitch in an eyelid for example, and thereby provide a clue.

Pioneering work was done in the 1960's by David Cheek and Leslie LeCron, published in their book *"Clinical Hypnotherapy,"* where, when working with a client, certain key areas were focused on, and in conjunction with a pendulum as a tool to detect an ideo-motor response, the subconscious mind could be accessed without having to use hypnosis.

A pendulum is a little weight in the form of a crystal or wooden cone, attached to a fine cord the end of which is held between two fingers. The pendulum can swing freely in response to the message it receives, either in a circular motion or back and forth or sideways. The person holding the pendulum does not initiate any movement, rather holds the pendulum very still and lets the energy move it. It is very easy to calibrate and use yourself. I regularly consult mine if I need to get an answer from my Inner Self.

In the mid-1980's sociologist Dr. Clark Cameron, and later Robert Detzler and his wife MaryAnn, further developed these key areas into specific charts to help clients address subconscious problems, and began teaching this method as it was showing such promising and lasting results. Detzler ended up founding the Spiritual Response Association (SRA) in 1991, and is the author of the book *"The Freedom Path"* (2006).

I find my SRT sessions immensely relaxing, as I lie stretched out on a massage table under a warm blanket while my practitioner "dowses", or moves, the pendulum over me. To be precise, she does not move it at all; my subconscious mind moves it as it reacts with her chart work and the questions she silently asks of me.

Ideomotor responses provide clues and she can address specific areas in my body and proceed to do clearing work of any negative energy or repeat programming that is causing an energy flow blockage. The purpose of this therapy is to restore harmony. I can emerge extremely relaxed or a little groggy as the clearing process sometimes takes a while to be completed. Afterwards, I feel a lot more energized, mentally focused and peaceful inside.

Recommended website:
https://spiritualresponse.com/

> **Recommended reading:**
>
> *"The Freedom Path"* (2006) by Robert E. Detzler
> *"Spiritual Healing"* (1998) by Robert E. Detzler

Biofeedback

According to the AAPB (The Association for Applied Psychophysiology and Biofeedback, Inc.) which is an international society for mind-body research, health care and education, biofeedback can be described as such:

> "Biofeedback is a process that enables an individual to learn how to change physiological activity for the purposes of improving health and performance. Precise instruments measure physiological activity such as brainwaves, heart function, breathing, muscle activity, and skin temperature. These instruments rapidly and accurately "feed-back" information to the user. The presentation of this information — often in conjunction with changes in thinking, emotions, and behavior — supports desired physiological changes. Over time, these changes can endure without continued use of an instrument."

Biofeedback is another way to access what is going on in the body in a non-invasive way, by using specific machines that become calibrated to your energetic field. It is a very relaxing experience as no action is required, while the practitioner does the "scanning" using a biofeedback instrument.

The recipient of biofeedback does not even have to be in the same room, this can be done remotely. Physiological as well as psycho-emotional imbalances can be addressed in this way, and changed over time as the ground work is laid for the body to function in a different way.

One area in which I used biofeedback was to clear chronic pain I experienced after my mastectomy and subsequent radiation therapy. What was fascinating was that I needed only a few sessions, and my body somehow found a new way of re-directing and self-correcting the underlying cause of the pain as it was taught how to do this. Not only did biofeedback bring me physical relief, it helped my body find its own path to deal with a physical imbalance. The pain dissolved over a period of a few months to the point of it being only a little uncomfortable at times. No pain medication was required anymore.

Depending on which location you have biofeedback therapy done you may be able to get it reimbursed through your health insurance (if in the US). I went for treatment in the office of a neuropsychologist. Initially my health insurance rejected the claims, however, when I appealed and showcased how much consistent chronic pain medication would add up to as opposed to a few biofeedback sessions, my claims were reconsidered. I see the efforts I took to appeal the initial rejection not necessarily as a nuisance, but as my role to play in the active re-education of our health care system.

Emotional Freedom Technique (EFT)

EFT is an easy-to-apply self-help technique that I find invaluable in moments where I need a so-called "quick-fix" such as a high stress or crisis management moment that can be a little overwhelming. I mainly use it in moments of emotional stress, but this technique can be applied to physical stressors and even chronic pain.

Also referred to as "tapping" all you do is use the tips of your fingers or the side of your hand to tap on certain key areas on your body, which correspond to certain meridian points. Meridians are based on the wisdom of ancient Traditional Chinese Medicine (TCM), and are energy lines on your body that connect various organs and allow your life force energy, or "chi" or "qi" to flow through.

The effect it has is that it helps me become centered again and more mindful about the task at hand. I feel more grounded and able to tackle the next step in a calmer way, despite it perhaps still being a rather hectic moment in my day.

Recommended websites:

http://www.emofree.com/
http://www.acos.org/articles/the-chinese-medi-cine-meridian-system/
http://www.thetappingsolution.com/what-is-eft-tap-ping/
http://eft.mercola.com/

Chiropractic Care via the Network Spinal Analysis Method

Ever since the birth of my son over eighteen years ago, I have made chiropractic care a part of my self-care healing regimen. I was introduced to it by a close friend when I complained of a stiff shoulder and back pain from hauling around the baby carrier. I have never looked back. It is invaluable for aligning my physical structure back into a pain-free place.

And then I was introduced to a more advanced type of chiropractic care that incorporates not only aligning your physical body, but also allowing your nervous system to autocorrect and self-adjust physical as well as emotional tension you did not even know you had, stuck in places that may be on opposite ends of where you are experiencing any symptoms: Network Spinal Analysis, combined with Somato Respiratory Integration, developed by Dr. Donald Epstein, DC. author of the book *"The Twelve Stages of Healing – A Network Approach to Wholeness" (1994)*.

Very gentle adjustments to the spine allow for the spontaneous release of any tension, be it physical, emotional or spiritual and support your brain to use existing tension as a fuel for involuntary spinal adjustments and self-corrections. The NSA / SRI chiropractor tunes into your body, guides it, and then the patient's body uses these suggestions to adjust itself through focused attention, gentle breathing and the free flow of movement that looks similar to wave-like motions when you are lying down on the table.

I learnt to fully get in touch with the rhythm of my body and experience the release of physical discomfort as well as emotional pain, both consciously as well as subconsciously. I leave feeling re-balanced and totally connected and aligned with my body, mind and spirit. Sometimes it takes a few hours for the processing to settle, depending on what was released, but I am shedding layer upon layer of unresolved issues that are often stuck deep within. All I need to do when lying down on the table is to give my body permission to go where it most needs to go on that particular day.

Recommended website:
https://wiseworldseminars.com/network-spinal-analysis

Recommended reading:
"The Twelve Stages of Healing–A Network Approach to Wholeness" (1994) by Donald M. Epstein, DC.

In conclusion, I want to make one point very clear; no matter which energy healing modalities we use, it does not prevent us from having to face life's challenges; we are still exposed to certain devastating lessons we need to learn. Emotions such as anger, fear, grief will still arise as we move through life. We won't simply feel happy and at peace all the time just because we are "clear". However, if our life energy can flow freely without blockages caused by stuck suppressed emotional trauma, whether we were aware that we had any or not, we are able to deal with these challenges and lessons much more easily.

There are many layers of unresolved issues we can address, but rather than this sounding overwhelming, understand that whatever needs to be taken care of to help you progress at that exact moment, will present itself to you. At that point, you will know what needs your attention. It would be contraindicated if we now started obsessively worrying about what other deep issues still need to be cleared, although we may feel there is still more to a particular situation. In that case, we can revisit this area with a few more sessions. It takes time to process what comes up, and we need to give our bodies and mind a chance to integrate.

As we move through life, bear in mind that experiencing all kinds of emotions is normal, but they are meant to flow through us, not get stuck and settle. It is essentially our job to try and release any negativity, or life-suppressing emotions whether at a conscious or subconscious level. And for that, we can gladly accept the help and guidance of a variety of techniques, a few of which I have outlined in this chapter. May this serve as the beginning of your emotional healing journey.

*In case you would like to start exploring, I have made it easy for you with my **START WITH ONE Guide** where I summarized all the references mentioned in this chapter Click here if you are reading a digital book version*

http://www.kirstinscancercare.com/start-one-guide/

or find it at

www.kirstinscancercare.com/awesomebookbonuses/

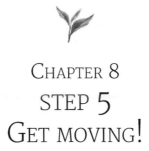

Chapter 8
Step 5
Get moving!

"To enjoy the glow to good health, you must exercise!"
Gene Tunney

If you were to ask me if I secretly struggled with any of the five steps I outline in this book, it would be this one! This book is, after all, about confessions...

Don't get me wrong, I do exercise and love the benefits I feel from it, but I am far from a regular gym-goer. In fact I have sunk hard-earned money into keeping my local gym afloat too many times to count.

You see, I love to be outside and walk, not jog, but walk at a jogger's pace, if that makes any sense. This is exactly how a friend of mine coined it when we would walk our dogs together in Munich, she jogging, I brisk-walking, both of us keeping the same pace. My dad calls it the "Kirstin stride."

Having to walk my dog, seeing him frolic outside, eager to

explore and sniff, gives me joy and motivates me to get out every day in most weather conditions. I love exercising in fresh air. I do not need to drown out any sounds around me with earphones, in fact I use this daily ritual to let my thoughts wander and dart into whatever direction they wish to go. The result is an exercised body, clarity of thought, a mapped-out To-Do list and creative content for my writing. And a happy, tired-out Max!

I also enjoy yoga, as it is something I can do at home as well as join a class to experience the energy and rhythm of yogis around me. I am always amazed at how much sweat stationary asanas, or yoga positions, can produce!

After my very first round of chemo, my husband and I took a slow walk along the fields and forests that surrounded Munich, and the house we were living in at the time. I could barely make it, having to stop every so often to rest, aghast at my lack of energy. I vividly remember wondering how on earth I would be able to tolerate this entire treatment. I felt crushed.

Movement was the best thing I could have done, and I felt better almost immediately after making it back home, quite the reverse of how I thought my day would unfold. One walk kicked my shocked system back into action, and I took note. With it came hope that maybe with a little resilience I would be able to make it through after all. I also noticed that on the days I exercised I slept better even during the notorious steroid-sleep-robbing days around each chemo treatment, the intensity and duration of my nausea improved and even the medication-induced con-stipation was more short-lived.

Granted, often the associated fatigue, pain and general uncom-fortable side effects may not exactly cause one to jump into action and start exercising. But even a little movement is better than not moving at all.

Mounting research is increasingly showing that some form of exercise, even if it's just very gentle movement, is exactly what will make cancer treatments more effective and the subsequently desired recovery faster.

A study completed almost twenty years ago on the effects of aerobic exercise on fatigue and psychological status of cancer patients during chemotherapy showed that those who partook in some form of aerobic exercise showed a marked reduction in fatigue and, in particular, fear and phobic anxiety.

I want to emphasize chronic fatigue, as this is by far the most common side effect experienced by most cancer patients undergoing traditional cancer treatment. It is often a vicious cycle, as treatments cause severe fatigue which makes many patients too weak to engage in any form of exercise, which leads to chronic inactivity, which leads to even more fatigue.

Exactly at this point exercise will help your body process the toxicity of treatments. Movement stimulates your lymphatic system, a major detox mechanism which relies on muscle contraction to pump the toxin and waste-products collecting lymphatic fluid through your body, channeling this to your organs of elimination. This system also plays a key role in boosting and regulating your immune function as it helps transport white blood cells throughout your body, helping to fight infections and offering repair and tissue regeneration.

Muscle wasting, or cachexia, can be both a symptom of cancer as well as associated with the effects of treatments, and is a condition which can be potentially life-threatening, especially when skeletal muscles are involved. These muscles, apart from enabling structural movement, have another very crucial function, that of protecting our internal organs.

Muscle wasting can occur as a result of cancer cells' ability to secrete inflammatory compounds that break down proteins making up muscle tissue. Treatments themselves are inflammatory and can cause this breakdown as well. Consistent inactivity can also lead to muscle shrinking. The problem is that once skeletal muscles begin to erode, so-called visceral proteins that make up your vital organs, begin to break down too. You want to keep skeletal muscles intact to ensure adequate protection of these vital organs.

Exercise can enhance long-term recovery and remission too, as a study published in the 2006 *Journal of Clinical Oncology* showed that linked exercise to the survival and decreased recurrence of stage 3 colon cancer patients. A further study concluded that just walking at an average pace of between three to five hours a week reduced the risk of death from breast cancer by up to 50%.

In a study, published in 2015, data was compared on the physical activity level and the risk of recurrence, or death, from breast cancer. Twenty-two different studies involving over 123,574 breast cancer patients over a follow-up period of between four and twelve years, showed that both pre-diagnosis and post-diagnosis exercise is an important intervention in enhancing the overall lifespan of breast cancer survivors.

What I find encouraging is that even if one was not that physically active before a diagnosis, but started including regular exercise post diagnosis, the risk factors are nevertheless significantly reduced.

Movement is a life-ensuring and life-promoting essential, one important outcome being the ability to oxygenate our cells. Remember cancer cannot survive in an oxygen-rich environment, and with exercise we can consistently contribute to this oxygenating environment.

In his comprehensive book *"Life Over Cancer"*, Dr. Keith Block, Director of the Block Center for Integrative Cancer Treatments in Illinois, makes a compelling case for including exercise as part of your physical care plan as it can directly affect cancer growth and proliferation.

Exercise can help reduce levels of growth-stimulating compounds such as excess estrogen, insulin and IGF-1 (insulin-like growth factor) and can increase the level of proteins in the blood that helps bind IGF-1 so it is less available.

Dr. Block cautions against both over-exercising and infrequent exercising, especially when you are not that fit, as this may subject the body to oxidative stress which can have a pro-cancer effect in your body.

Why a good night's sleep is vitally important for you

It may surprise you to learn that there is another component to overall fitness which is the exact opposite of physical activity, however equally as important, and that is getting sufficient rest and sleep!

According to Dr. Block, studies have shown that patients with few side effects but interrupted sleep patterns felt worse and reported a poorer quality of life than patients with more severe side effects but regular sleep patterns.

The core fitness plan at the Block Center for Integrative Cancer Treatments concurs that these two phases, the rest phase and the activity phase, contribute equally to overall fitness, and are mutually enhancing: good quality sleep will help you exercise, and exercise will help you sleep.

Perhaps, you have the best intentions to exercise, but wind up in a self-defeating cycle of feeling extremely lethargic, needing naps during the day to function at all, frequently waking up during the night and then feeling exhausted in the morning which easily lasts throughout the day.

You may be experiencing an interrupted circadian rhythm. The National Institute of General Medical Sciences (NIGMS) defines the circadian rhythm as "physical, mental and behavioral changes that follow a roughly 24-hour cycle, responding primarily to light and darkness in an organism's environment". These organisms are not just limited to humans, they also include animals, plants and many tiny microbes. In fact all living beings use this rhythm to adjust to the earth's rotation around its axis.

The circadian rhythm is not to be underestimated. It not only can influence sleep-wake cycles, but also the release of hormones, body temperature fluctuations and other important bodily functions. An imbalanced circadian rhythm has been linked to various sleep disorders, including those resulting from jet lag, but also to other health issues such as obesity, diabetes, depression and cancer.

Groups of cells within our body, our so-called biological clock, control our individual circadian rhythm. The "master clock" (called the suprachiasmatic nucleus, or SCN) is a group of about 20,000 nerve cells located in the hypothalamus, an area of the brain just behind your eyes. They respond mainly to light, and are responsible for producing the hormone melatonin to make you sleepy and groggy.

In 2007, the International Agency for Research on Cancer (IARC) classified "shiftwork that involves circadian disruption as ***probably carcinogenic to humans***". That particular study looked at the possible relationship between disruptions of normal circadian rhythms and genetic mutations driving cancer cells. The aim was to isolate potential causes such as exposure to light at night and sleep disruption, when considering targeted anti-cancer therapies.

A 2012 review of existing studies, published in the Journal of Molecular Medicine, once again analyzed whether disruptions in circadian rhythms had any effect on possible cancer growth.

The review looked at whether these disruptions had an impact on various stages of cancer development, such as genetic mutations, tumor growth and proliferation, angiogenesis (blood vessel supply to the tumor), apoptosis (programmed cell death) and response to hormone receptors. They concluded that "a major consequence of modern lifestyle is disruption of circadian rhythms. Circadian disruptions induced by light at night, genetic or epigenetic variations in circadian genes and interactions between genes and environment form a set of data that propose that some cancer cases could be explained by these mechanisms".

I notice almost immediately if I did not get sufficient sleep, in my case that just needs to be two or three consecutive days of either too little or very disrupted sleep. It not only affects my energy levels, but also my psyche. I am less motivated, less focused and far less convinced that I am capable of achieving what needs to be done. Crisis management during that time is far less effective than when I am fully refreshed from enough sleep. I am sure most, if not all, of you reading this can fully relate.

Almost weekly, a client will ask me whether I can recommend any supplement to take that will help combat some form of insomnia, besides relying on prescription anti-depressants or sleep aids. I always begin by asking a couple of questions, as the underlying reasons can be so diverse, but need to be taken into consideration.

This is a self-defeating cycle of imbalance that we can find ourselves in, and wonder why our bodies are self-sabotaging themselves. We get to bed too late, but wake up way too early and are fully alert, knowing full well that we did not have enough sleep.

Alternatively, we repeatedly wake up only to find our minds racing ahead and bombarding us with our current worries, or even the To-Do list, both of which seem to grow much more menacing in the middle of the night than during the day.

Sometimes we drank that glass of water too late, or our bladders are affected by a particular chemo drug, either way that need to go pee, will beat any mindful intention to simply ignore and go back to sleep.

I won't even start on the hot flash – night sweat topic, which, as many of you know, can become a pretty intimate companion for us pre or full-blown post-menopausal women, especially if it is chemo or hormone treatment induced.

And at other times, we are trying to digest the news that we, or a loved one, has received a potentially life-threatening diagnosis, a kind of stress that can kick-start a period of severe anxiety with chronic insomnia as a nightly companion.

On a lighter note, if the fact that you are unable to convince your teenager to go to sleep before 11-12 pm is causing you sleepless nights, studies have shown that this is due to a naturally occurring shift in their circadian rhythms at this time in their lives.

The National Sleep Foundation refers to this as a "sleep phase delay". The problem is that here in the US the start times of some high schools requires them to leave the house between 6 and 6:30 am. This can make it difficult for them to get the sleep they need. The so-called morning circadian dip, usually between 3:00-7:00 am, can thus be even longer if they didn't get sufficient sleep, and may last until 9:00 or 10:00 am, placing the retention capability of the first few school lessons into question.

For years, I was frustrated at the frequency with which my daughter would get sick each year between November and March. I thought it coincided with winter in New Jersey, until I saw a pattern in her lack of adequate sleep and strength of her immune system. For her, enough sleep is the single most defining factor in how strong her immunity is when it comes to fighting off infections she is exposed to.

Each reason, and there may be others besides the ones I listed above, requires a slightly different approach, and while there are certain targeted supplement protocols that can definitely make a difference, we also need to think beyond the popping a pill remedy if we wish to regain a restorative sleep pattern.

Here are a few things that I regularly implement myself and have had the most success with, depending on my underlying reason for intermittent insomnia:

- Our bedroom is a sleep-enhancing sanctuary. We keep distractions to a minimum, which means no screens, no electrical appliances besides bedside lamps. Even our alarm clock is battery-driven to reduce exposure to EMFs and so-called "dirty" electricity (refer to a previous chapter on reducing toxicity).

- I avoid coffee or green tea caffeine in the evening.

- I try and stick to a regular day schedule as this can normalize my body's circadian rhythm. I try and go to bed and get up around the same time each day. Weekends are slightly adjusted.

- I have developed a relaxing night time routine. No computer screen work in the last hour before bedtime, it makes a huge difference for me!

- We sleep in complete darkness. No night lights, no flashing alarm clocks. I even remove the electric toothbrush from its charger as that flashing light from the bathroom can illuminate our entire bedroom.

- I aim to make sleep the most important priority for the majority of the time, meaning I intentionally don't get distracted by working late, watching a late movie, answering emails or checking Facebook before bedtime.

- I make sure I get a minimum of 30 minutes of bright daylight exposure per day. Sunshine signals to the brain to stop producing the sleep hormone melatonin. If I work from home, my blinds are up on an overcast day and my LED or daylight lights are on.

- I avoid large meals close to my bed time. I eat at least three to four hours before going to bed. On nights where we do end up having to eat later, I make sure I eat a small portion and leave room, meaning I am not fully satiated, but enough to avoid a growling stomach or blood sugar dip. Fruit eaten on its own will digest within 15 to 40 minutes, so if I am peckish because the evening extends longer than usual, I may have an apple or a banana.

- I have developed a balanced exercise program consisting of some aerobic exercise combined with more gentle as well as meditative forms of movement.

BREATHING ESSENTIALS

Another aspect of fitness and overall movement, besides good sleep, which also has a direct effect on everyday activity as well as being an important cancer-fighting strategy, is proper breathing.

Many of us simply fail to take deep, restorative breaths, focusing rather on shallow or chest breathing. Often we even breathe irregularly or hold our breath without noticing. This fills only the top part of our lungs, and has a much more far-reaching consequence as it does not properly oxygenate our blood!

As a Harvard Mental Health Letter (2009) mentioned, "shallow breathing hobbles the diaphragm's range of motion". The result is that a large group of small blood vessels in the lower parts of your lungs, are never exposed to fully oxygenated air, leaving you short-breathed, light-headed and often feeling claustrophobic.

Oxygen shortage can show up in the form of many other symptoms too, such as high blood pressure, poor memory or concentration, anxiety and muscle spasms. Remember cancer cells prefer an anaerobic (low-oxygenated) environment.

Here's a quick breathing exercise you can do right now while you are reading this to illustrate the difference between shallow chest breathing, and deep abdominal or belly breathing.

1. You want to bring air down to the bottom of your lungs, using your diaphragm, which is a sheet of muscle intended for enabling us to engage in deep breathing.

2. Create more space for your lungs to expand when breathing downwards, make sure you don't hunch your shoulders.

3. Put your hands on your belly, take a deep breath and feel the air travel in through your nose, fully expanding your lungs with rich, oxygenated air, pressing the diaphragm down and allowing your belly to rise. You actually want to see that belly protrude outwards.

4. As you exhale, sink your belly back down and lift your diaphragm upwards, pressing against the lungs to expel carbon-dioxide-rich air.

5. Do this a few times and then resume your normal breathing. Keep in mind that throughout the day, you

want to take a few minutes a couple of times and practice deep belly breathing.

I have consciously taught myself to practice this deep breathing fairly frequently during the day, and have found that over the years, my body almost instantly falls into an ecstatic pattern of gratitude as it welcomes the true breath of fresh air. As a result of the Network Spinal Analysis (NSA) entrainments I receive at my chiropractor's office on a weekly basis, I have noticed that occasionally my body is so eager to embrace this deep breathing that it involuntarily releases any tension by sending gentle waves through my spine.

I use this to my advantage on a sleepless night when I wake up and have trouble falling back asleep right away. Sometimes a hot flash wakes me, sometimes it's the deadline I am trying to meet or a family issue, but this type of deep breathing, coupled with my NSA work, usually does the trick as it instantly relaxes my entire body and I don't even notice as I drift off to sleep again.

My supplement regimen includes magnesium, which I take every night, sometimes in combination with the amino acid GABA (gamma-aminobutyric acid). Both help induce a state of calm and contribute to a natural state of relaxation that in my, and my husband's case, can be felt almost within the hour of taking both together.

EXERCISE ESSENTIALS

Become aware of your posture

Many of us have issues with poor posture these days. Just think of how we all hunch over our screens, shoulders drooping, spine all scrunched up, and then we wonder why our entire back hurts.

After my bilateral mastectomy, I invariably wanted to protect that area even after the initial pain from surgery subsided. I did not notice how I was bending over my shoulders. The result was strong muscle tension radiating from the back of my neck all the way down to my lower back, causing me almost daily headaches and a chronically disrupted sleep pattern.

Once I became aware of what I was doing, I consciously started to pay attention to straightening my shoulders and upper torso, a few times a day. The tension slowly subsided over the next few weeks. I did, however, need to intervene with the help of bio-feedback and chiropractic care to "re-train" my muscles into identifying what is a normal state for them to be in.

From that time on, checking in every so often with my posture has become one of the easiest self-care practices I can do, any-where, anytime. Yoga or Pilates of course can also help you con-nect with your own body and identify which muscle groups you can manipulate and stretch to regain a posture that is ideal for your body composition.

Use your core abdominal muscles

At the risk of sounding like my yoga instructor, I cannot empha-size enough how important it is to become aware of, and engage, your core abdominal muscles. They provide the backbone for good posture, they essentially carry your body, they massage our internal organs and help encourage a smooth digestive process. While core muscle work is an integral part of yoga, pilates, certain gym machines and live exercise classes, what I love is the fact that you can work on these muscle groups even if you are bedridden.

Simply start right now by first identifying this muscle group: lie on your back, in bed or on the floor, with your knees bent

and both feet planted on the ground. Your lower back will be up in the air, leaving a little hollow gap. Breathe in, and when breathing out, gently press your lower back into the floor, closing that gap, but don't use your buttocks to help you.

These are your core abdominal muscles, the ones you can feel when you tighten your stomach muscles and use your finger to prod to see how much resistance there is, despite some possible belly blubber in that area.

You can easily exercise them daily following the above instructions, no need to always lie on the floor or in bed, try this while driving or standing in line somewhere. Yes, this is a form of exercise, so credit it accordingly, and when you look at it this way, suddenly you do have enough time in your day to do it.

WHOLE BODY EXERCISES

Stretching Exercises

There are numerous benefits to stretching on a regular basis, including increased flexibility of various muscles and associated joints, a greater range of motion, overall body awareness, much quicker recovery after surgery and of course supporting the lymphatic system.

Bear in mind that not just muscles get stretched, but also surrounding connective tissues. You feel the effects of inadequate stretching if you at times experience pain or discomfort during or after exercising. A tightening of these surrounding tissues can be the underlying cause.

An ideal frequency for receiving the full benefits of stretching is to do it for ten to fifteen minutes every day. Alternatively, if you manage to stretch for just five minutes at a time, but do it three times per day, you will experience the comfort of a stretched body. I bet you can fit this into your day somewhere.

Why not try a quick stretch now?

Lengthen your neck by reaching for the ceiling with the crown of your head. At the same time bring your shoulder blades together towards the center of your back and move them slightly down. This is called complementary opposition, and is a standard principle in many yoga positions. Even though you may not be thinking of this as a form of exercise as it requires such minimal overall movement, you are lengthening and stretching your neck muscles. Easy, isn't it? Besides yoga, other modalities that heavily rely on this technique are pilates, tai chi and qi gong.

Gentle stretching becomes even more important after surgery, once the initial wound has healed and you have the approval by your surgeon. I recommend you ask very specifically to what extent you may stretch the surgical area so that you know what will be a normal reaction as there will be pain and discomfort in the beginning. This is due to nerves having being severed and the swelling associated with the body's natural healing process. You will obviously want to have a scale at which you know something is not right.

One of my clients was experiencing pain after her chemotherapy port-a-cath, a catheter with a port inserted into a vein to administer treatment, was surgically inserted. She received her first infusion the same day, a practice I would discourage as you want the site to heal a little before starting with the rigorous chemo treatments. She began gentle stretching exercises, but the pain did not subside. She initially thought it was due to this overwhelm effect, however, as it turned out, she had a blood clot, and ended up having to have her port removed in an emergency surgery.

Strengthening Exercises

The main benefits of strengthening exercises are improving your lean muscle mass, improving musculoskeletal strength, and supporting bone density. The aim is not necessarily to bulk up, but to increase overall muscle strength using mainly weight bearing exercises and some form of resistance training.

You want to focus on training different muscle groups in a rotational way so that they can recover from the previous exercise, which can be seen as some form of oxidative stress.

Ideally, a strengthening program focuses on eight to ten different exercises performed at a number of repetitions each. It is important to warm up and stretch before and after to prevent any undue stress on tissue and ligaments. It is important here too to engage your core abdominal muscles and to breathe deeply throughout the exercise routine.

You do not need to join a gym to have access to strengthening exercise machines. As a start, you can have a selection of the following exercise tools at home:

- Thera-band stretch bands

- Stability balls

- Resistance cords

I suggest you google any of these terms, or find them in Amazon. com. Next you google related exercises, and there are a plethora of options on YouTube for you to follow for free, or for a nominal membership fee, it all depends on whom you connect with, it is a personal affinity decision you need to make. You may click with some instructors, but not others.

I remember using a Yogalates DVD at home, and my husband could not stand the voice of the instructor, whereas I loved the types of exercises she offered and how she talked you through them so you did not have to watch the screen all the time, craning your neck while you were trying to follow along. That made up for the a little too velvety voice.

If going to the gym, or joining a live class is not an option for you, make a date with your computer and spend an evening sifting through Google and YouTube to find a guided exercise program that you connect with. Next, decide on a regular time, and place, at home to engage in your own personalized exercise routine, and make it an appointment on your calendar.

If, on the other hand, you need the vibrancy and the companionship of people around you, I challenge you now to find a local gym, whether it is a large facility or a smaller, more personalized one that seem to pop up everywhere now, or any other exercise class you connect with. If you have a friend who will do this with you, great, but bear in mind that you may find a new one in that exercise class you just joined.

There are a plethora of classes for cancer patients and survivors offered almost everywhere these days, and this is a gentle way of approaching a regular strengthening exercise regimen.

AEROBIC AND ENDURANCE EXERCISES

This is by far the best form of exercise to increase oxygen levels in your blood and to your cells, improve heart and lung function and to support your lymph flow. Make sure all surgery sites are fully healed before you engage in any of the more rigorous exercises mentioned below.

The sky's the limit here when it comes to options: walking, swimming, jogging, biking, stair-climbing, treadmill, any sports such as tennis, basketball, volleyball, even dancing, anything that gets your heart rate up and pounding. Even here you have at home options, and my favorite one is the portable indoor trampoline rebounder.

The history of the rebounder is quite interesting. In the 1980's NASA was trying to figure out a way to help astronauts recover and regain bone and muscle mass after being in space.

A gravity-based exercise like hopping (not jumping) on the rebounder makes use of an increased G-force action, which can increase bone mass. Also, each cell in the body has to respond to the acceleration and deceleration of the up and down motion. This is also beneficial for the lymphatic system which transports immune cells throughout the body and collects and carries away waste and toxins.

Keep in mind how effective hopping on a rebounder can be for you. As this is indoors, all you want to do is use the balls of your feet and move up and down in a hopping motion, your foot does not fully lift off the mat. An ideal time span to exercise is between twenty to thirty minutes three to four times per week, unless you combine it with another form of aerobic exercise.

Interval training is an important aspect to consider with any aerobic style exercise. The aim here is to increase as well as decrease your heart rate as quickly as you can. This trains your cardiac system to deal with stress and be able to return to its normal state fairly rapidly. A healthy heart can slow down much faster than a compromised heart.

Several cancer treatment drugs can damage your heart health, so for those of us affected by this, myself included as I received the targeted antibody treatment Herceptin for a total of two years, it is imperative that we practice this exercise, also called "cardiac recovery conditioning", as regularly as we can to get our hearts back in shape.

This type of exercise is best done in sets. One set, for example constitutes five minutes of aerobic activity followed by 10 minutes rest. Do about 5 such sets a day if possible.

I include my aerobics when I walk our dog Max. I speed up my walking and pump my arms, very similar to power walking that used to be all the rage a few years ago. Bottom line, it looks a bit funny, but does the trick in getting my heart to race and me out of breath. Then I slow down a little to a normal paced walking stride. If I wanted to I could even break out into a jog, and then walk in between.

What if you are not an exercise friend?

I still recommend you find something that works for you, and start with shorter periods a day, or every other day, just to get into the rhythm and flow of regular exercise. It is important to include all five styles of exercise discussed: posture, core muscles, stretching, strengthening and aerobic or endurance training.

It also depends on where you are at in your cancer journey. If you are in the middle of your cancer treatments, you just want to make sure you get anything in, and the extent will largely depend on how actively involved and fit you were before your treatments.

This is not the ideal time to start all out with a new exercise regimen. If, however, you are done with your treatments, your focus will be on getting your pre-treatment strength and endurance back at first, then making sure you maintain an ideal healthy weight based on your physique. Exercise for losing excess weight should involve more endurance/aerobic type as well as strength training to increase muscle mass. Muscles burn more calories than fat.

I understand repetition can become boring, and I tend to fall into the category of becoming bored easily, unless I am outside exercising with Max. Somehow, no single day is the same as nature will present itself slightly differently each day, and that is what attracts me personally to being outside. I also bike ride recreationally with my husband on weekends if our family time allows, or we take Max on extended hikes.

I have a variety of indoor options at home that include a range of different DVDs or YouTube clips, again to offer myself variety. If I use the indoor elliptical trainer I always watch a German documentary to keep my mind off the actual exercise regimen, and keep up with my German, nothing like multi-tasking!

Full body massage

You may not associate a full body massage with a topic on movement, but I include all kinds of movement including the type that happens on a cellular level.

If you have healed from surgery, do not have an existing malignant tumor site or fully diagnosed lymphedema, a full body massage has a range of benefits such as helping to oxygenate tissues and organs, improving circulation to stimulate lymph flow, stimulating natural killer (NK) cell production, helping with flexibility and range of motion as well as being a great rehabilitation tool after surgery to reduce pain and swelling.

A Study on the effect of therapeutic massage was done with patients treated at the Memorial Sloan–Kettering Cancer Center in New York City. That study evaluated changes in pain, fatigue, stress and anxiety, nausea, and depression after receiving some form of massage.

Participants included 1,290 cancer patients and 12 licensed massage therapists. Patients selected among three different massage styles: Swedish, light touch, and foot massage. Researchers noted a decline in the severity of symptoms by about 50%, although the effects of massage were short-term, indicating that regular sessions offered a longer-term benefit.

Anxiety on its own, particularly procedural anxiety before radiation therapy was significantly reduced, by as much as 43%.

Researchers concluded that *"the effects (of manipulation of body tissues and corresponding relief from a broad range of symptoms) are distributed, and reciprocal interplay between the body and mind is evident. We have literally just "touched" the surface of meridian research, but the meridian system appears to be an important communication link between myofascial tissue and the nervous system. The implications for symptom control in cancer patients are important, opening up new research avenues that link self-reported pain with the subjective quality of suffering. The reciprocal body–mind relationship and its manipulation is an important target for therapies that can reduce suffering".*

From personal experience, receiving a massage is a little piece of heaven, a blessing in disguise. Once you have had one, you know why dogs, when scratched, contort their bodies in absolute bliss into quite comical positions, totally oblivious to how hilarious they look. Their way of succumbing to a massage, not quite ours, but you get the drift. Apart from deeply relaxing, I feel fully invigorated and alive afterward, aware of a pulsating vibe that is, essentially, me.

Besides full body massages, I have also experienced two other massage modalities, both lymphatic drainage massages as well as craniosacral therapy.

Lymphatic drainage massage is a gentle, surface-touch, rhythmic massage that helps move lymph fluid throughout the lymphatic vessels that are spread through the body much like our expansive system of blood vessels. It helps reduce edema (swelling) and aids in removing toxins and cellular waste material.

After my bilateral mastectomy, in which lymph nodes were also removed under my arm, I began feeling a tightness in my right arm, although no swelling was visible yet. I suspected I might have lymphedema, which is a swelling due to accumulated lymph fluid that cannot flow as easily because of a disruption in the lymphatic system, usually as a result of surgical removal of lymph nodes.

I immediately utilized the rehabilitation services at the hospital and saw a physical therapist, certified in lymphatic drainage massage, who showed me how I could apply this gentle yet very effective technique at home.

Luckily, after a few sessions, regular at home applications and wearing a compression arm stocking for a few weeks, the feeling subsided and it was not considered full blown lymphedema, a condition which is permanent.

To this day I am very mindful of not aggravating this arm, which I did one Spring when I was filling all our outside pots on our deck with bright annuals. I don't carry a potting soil bag anymore, but I did lift it up a little to decant the soil into the pot. Bad idea! Similar tightness again, and this has become my warning sign that I need to back off. No more heavy lifting. A little self-massage usually calms everything down again. Every time I fly I wear my compression stocking as the change in altitude seems to trigger a similar reaction.

Craniosacral therapy is another form of a gentle, hands-on approach that releases deep-seated tension in the membranes and fluid, the so-called craniosacral system, along with the spine and brain. It restores balance to the cranial-sacral system, which in turn enhances a natural healing process, relieves pain, and strengthens the central nervous system.

Stress and strain can cause the body tissues to distort the craniosacral system which, in turn, can affect the central nervous system. A CST practitioner can feel these distortions through tapping into the rhythm of the fluid pulsating around the spinal cord and brain, and with gentle touch adjustments can help the body self-correct these imbalances.

It is an incredibly relaxing experience, and can sometimes also lead to the release of suppressed emotions as the body gently releases any stuck energy.

In concluding this chapter on exercise and getting moving, I wanted to briefly mention the importance of maintaining a healthy weight to prevent a possible cancer recurrence, and help our body stay on track.

I would like to reference a collaborative global study, published in 2016 that looked at the relationship between the growing, and by now global, obesity epidemic and overall mortality rate across various cultures.

This meta-analysis, which looked at the results of 239 different published studies, was a joint venture funded by the US National Institutes of Health, the UK Medical Research Council, the British Heart Foundation, and the National Institute for Health Research, and included over 10 million participants from Asia, Australia, New Zealand, Europe, and North America.

It concluded that there was indeed a link between obesity and higher mortality rates across all nations studied, highlighting the fact that being overweight has a direct influence on your health no matter your genetic background, dietary habits, climate conditions, culture or lifestyle factors.

Nowadays, it is fairly easy to become even a little overweight as our sedentary lifestyles, the overall lack of proper sleep, convenient rather than nutrient-dense driven dietary habits and high levels of poorly managed stress exposure, can set our bodies up for a chronic struggle to maintain a health-enforcing balance.

Measuring tools such as the Body Mass Index (BMI), devised by the World Health Organization (WHO) to measure the ratio of body fat to overall body weight, have been used worldwide for decades and give people a measure of whether or not they fall into the normal range of between 18.5 and 25.

Google BMI calculator and you will have access to a host of conversion tools to get your reading instantly. However, new evidence is surfacing that the BMI alone may not be all there is to it when it comes to controlling your body weight.

The BMI reading can disadvantage people that have denser bone structure, but happen to be metabolically healthy, despite having a higher BMI. A study published in 2016 concluded that in the US over 70 million people with BMI readings are misclassified as being either cardio-metabolically unhealthy or even cardio-metabolically healthy. Over 30% of people with normal weight were in fact cardio-metabolically unhealthy. They concluded that relying solely on BMI readings as a health risk assessment is inadequate, and sometimes misleading.

While researching this I came across a website by a German scientific author, Christian Bachmann. In 2014, in collaboration with the University of Zurich Institute of Social and Preventive Medicine, Bachmann used data gathered from a life expectancy calculator to come up with what he calls the SBMI, the Smart Body Mass Index. Essentially, it is a different calculating tool that does take into account age, gender, where in the body fat is actually stored, and what the health implications of this fat location mean for your overall risk assessment.

I did not come across evidence-based research to determine the validity of this tool to provide a more accurate health risk assessment, but I thought his rationale for developing the SBMI made some sense, and felt like sharing it here, for interest sake.

I cannot end this chapter without mentioning calorie counting. While this may be helpful as a tool when trying to prevent treatment-induced weight loss (cachexia), I do not like applying it as a weight management technique. Way too many calorie-counting diet programs have turned a calorie into something we need to be wary of, that can make us gain weight or prevent us from losing it. It is true that if we eat more calories than we can burn, the excess calories will be deposited as fat.

However, it fails to consider two important points: calories have a nutritional value, and not all calories are thus equal. And the rate at which a calorie is burned into energy in our body varies depending on some important factors that are unique to each of us, and that are, mostly, within our control.

Not all calories are equal

Calories have a nutritional value beyond providing you with energy. Compare a bunch of fresh, raw broccoli to a plate of packaged chips. Each can have equal amounts of calories. However, the calories you obtain from broccoli nourish and feed your body with vital nutrients, while the calories from chips are obtained mainly from hydrogenated fats and refined sugar.

Not only are these empty calories, but they also deplete your body of vital nutrients, which leads to an undernourished body and potential resultant food cravings. They also can slow down your metabolism, dysregulate your hormones and switch on your fat-storing mode.

Jonathan Bailor in his book *"The Calorie Myth: How to Eat More,*

Exercise Less, Lose Weight and Live Better," elaborates on how sugar, starches, processed fats, and other poor-quality foods, affect the ability of our hormones to regulate our metabolism. The problem we struggle with when trying to lose weight isn't because we are eating too many calories, it's eating the wrong foods! Understand that food has a complex effect on your body, and cannot be reduced to a simplified counting tool. You need to look at what's on your plate.

You can control how effectively calories are used in your body

It makes no real sense to zone in on weight management by measuring calories alone. Each individual has a different rate of metabolism, meaning each of us burns calories in a different way. We have different caloric needs depending on certain factors unique to us and our lifestyles, beginning with our age and gender. Men burn more calories than women as they have less body fat and more muscle, and this is why women need to focus on more weight-bearing exercises to burn more calories. Other factors include our inherited metabolic type, the physical condition of our body, eating the wrong foods, and how much stress we are exposed to.

In short, what we feed our bodies, how much we move them, what our current weight is and how we deal with stress, all has an effect on how efficiently calories are burned to energy in our bodies.

Rather than analyzing each mouthful according to its caloric value, focus on eating nutrient-dense and fiber-rich foods, avoid empty calories (from refined foods and sweet drinks), and exercise portion control. When you eat out, just because a restaurant chef dolls out a portion size you can feed half an army on, does not mean you need to comply and eat it.

Let's remain mindful that measuring tools are just numbers in the end, but are not the all-defining road map determining which exact path we need to follow to achieve and maintain our ideal weight.

Similarly, exercise is relative and we each may prefer different styles and intensities. It is important to remember that some form of movement needs to be an integral part of your overall health and wellness plan. Just start with something, and let that be your foundation upon which to build your regular movement plan.

Why not start now? Here is my basic
KEEPING IN SHAPE Quick-Start Guide
Click here if you are reading a digital book version

http://www.kirstinscancercare.com/keeping-shape-quickstart-guide/

or find it at
www.kirstinscancercare.com/awesomebookbonuses/

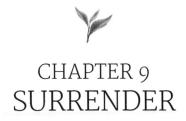

CHAPTER 9
SURRENDER

"We must let go of the life we have planned, so as to accept
the one that is waiting for us."
Joseph Campbell

When I was a girl I had visions of what my life would be like when I was all grown up. To a large extent it was based on what I wanted to see changed in my immediate surroundings.

As I was an only child, I wanted a larger family. In dreams I saw I would have two children, a boy and a girl. It is strange how these recurrent dreams would always show an older boy and a younger girl, which is exactly what I was blessed with when becoming a mother.

Life would also allow me to experience the loss of two conceived fetuses in between my children, not something in my original vision or dream.

My mother refused to learn how to drive a car, personal insecurities and fear from her experience associated with a car accident she was involved in as a young woman kept her entrapped, and she chose not to release this lingering trauma. This meant that in a country like South Africa with no public transportation, she was totally dependent on being driven around. She was frustrated and often resentful as a result of this lack of independent mobility. I made sure I passed my driver's license exam on the day of my 18th birthday.

Visions of being a fiercely independent and self-sufficient woman dominated my early twenties as I first attended University, then graduate business school, started a career at an educational institution, and moved in with my now husband for two years before marriage to "test" the waters before committing to the long haul. For us that translates into 24 years now and still going strong.

I had our first child in my late twenties, when we were ready to start a family. I made a choice to stay at home with our little family initially and forego a continuous career, planning to re-enter the workforce once the kids were ready for pre-school as I wanted to be fully present as a mother when they were toddlers.

Things in my life were happening as planned. I had managed to live up to my vision up until that point, confident I was carving my way through the jungle of life, accepting certain inevitable bumps in the road.

We don't make room for life-altering challenges, even though we know they will present themselves. When they do happen and rattle forcefully at the cage we call our life-so-far, we are still shocked that it's "our turn". We then either choose to re-design our vision and pro-actively tackle it head on, or stay in a passive-reactive mode as we fumble our way through it and cling to a fading image.

I have done both. The passive reactive mode led me down a rabbit hole of lingering, and compounding, discontent and disrespect towards myself that only surfaced when I was confronting the root causes of my cancers. Fumbling along was no longer an option, and I needed to face my own visions and dreams and understand that what I had neglected the most was an awareness of the fluidity of life, the role I played in getting me to the point where I was at, and who this Kirstin I saw reflected in a mirror really was.

This can easily be misconstrued as a blame-game, which is not at all what I am referring to. We make our choices to the best of our knowledge and ability at the time, and looking back on them from a wiser perspective, need to honor that without judgment.

When we become aware, and look back, we will inevitably see signs we missed that were way pointers for us and could have enabled us to make different decisions. The only purpose of doing this is to serve as a guide moving forward, as we internalize this awakened awareness and apply it with honesty and transparency to our lives.

I needed to confront my emotional baggage, the known as well as what was hidden in the depths of my subconscious that was gluing me to the spot, just as I needed to be honest with myself. I had to own up that I needed to spread my wings beyond home and motherhood, and become immersed and engaged again in a much broader environment where I could fully utilize what I was capable of doing. There was so much more I could give and contribute, and not pursuing this was consuming me from the inside.

I also needed to break free of the main restraint that was holding me back, and I am sure many of you can resonate with what I am going to say now. "What if I get cancer again? Despite all that I do." Here I am, teaching and empowering fellow cancer warriors to reclaim their lives by systematically incorporating lifestyle changes in five crucial areas of healing, but what if that is not enough?

I came to the humble realization that there is no judge to determine what exactly is enough. I am on my life path, and I do not see the full length of it ahead of me, nor what obstacles I may still face. What matters the most is what I do with my life right now, and I do take full ownership of steering my own ship.

I am not afraid of death, having come face-to-face with it on numerous hypnotherapy journeys. Of course I still want to give my current life all I have, engage wholeheartedly and passionately with all the people closest to me, and those that are yet to find me, for there is a reason we are all together at this moment in time. But I have learnt to surrender and let go of exact expectations, and at times am still learning this, as it, like so many other things, is a process.

This does not mean I sit back and let life happen, waiting for what will come my way. I am actively involved in navigating my way, living my 5 Step Process consciously, and with full intention, every single day. I monitor my health with the help of a team of integrative doctors and holistic practitioners just as I provide this guidance to my clients. I fully respect and incorporate conventional medicine for the value it can add, but true healing transcends its current boundaries. Starting with the limited follow-up tests on offer, I look elsewhere and tap into the myriad of resources a functional medical approach has to offer.

It was, and still is, my own choice to transform the relationship I had with cancer, embracing this physical, mental and emotional imbalance for what it was, a lesson in my life, meant to be understood and re-calibrated through conscious awareness of who we really are, what powers we each have and that we just need to show up for ourselves.

I hope I have given you a new perspective on how you too can transform your relationship with cancer when incorporating the 5 Step Process into your own life. You are meant to soar above this challenge and view it for what it truly is, a life altering opportunity to re-connect with yourself and consciously live your life's purpose.

****

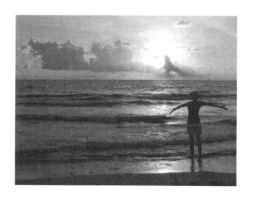

To connect with Kirstin to find out how she can
guide you to begin your own transformation journey,
visit her at www.kirstinscancercare.com
or email: kirstin@kirstinscancercare.com

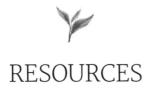

RESOURCES

DOWNLOADABLE CHEAT SHEETS

Click here or find them at www.kirstinscancercare.com/awesomebookbonuses/

1. BALANCE YOUR BLOOD SUGAR Cheat Sheet
   http://www.kirstinscancercare.com/balance-blood-sugar-cheat-sheet/

2. CLEAN PRODUCTS Cheat Sheet
   http://www.kirstinscancercare.com/clean-products-cheat-sheet/

3. 3 STEPS TO RETRAIN YOUR BRAIN Worksheet
   http://www.kirstinscancercare.com/3-steps-retrain-brain-worksheet/

4. START WITH ONE Guide
   http://www.kirstinscancercare.com/start-one-guide/

5. KEEPING IN SHAPE Quickstart Guide
   http://www.kirstinscancercare.com/keeping-shape-quickstart-guide/

Animal Welfare Approved (animalwelfareapproved.org)

Certifiedhumane.org

Monterey Bay Aquarium Seafood Watch (seafoodwatch.org)

Center for Food Safety (centerforfoodsafety.org)

Natural Food Coloring: www.colorgarden.net (US), www.ddw-color.com (EU)

Environmental Working Group (ewg.org)

"Rethinking Cancer" by EWG (ewg.org/cancer)

Food and Water Watch (foodandwaterwatch.org)
Just Label It (justlabelit.org)

Non-GMO Project (nongmoproject.org)

TED Talks
What's wrong with what we eat by Mark Bittman, NY Times Food Writer.

FOOD MOVIES
- Forksoverknives.com (great recipes!)

- Food Inc.

Center for Science in the Public Interest (CSPI) (cspinet.org)

"Zapped! Irradiation & the Death of Food" by Winonah Hauter & Mark Worth.

"What the Fork are you eating? An Action Plan for your Pantry and Plate" by Stefanie Sacks.

"The Safe Shopper's Bible: A Consumer's Guide to Nontoxic Household Products, Cosmetics, and Food" by David Steinman and Samuel S. Epstein, MD.

"Zapped: Why Your Cell Phone Shouldn't Be Your Alarm Clock and 1268 Ways to Outsamrt the hazards of Electronic Pollution" by Ann Louise Gittleman (2010) Harper Collins Publishers.

"Dirty Electricity: Electrification and the Diseases of Civilization" by Samuel Milham MD MPH (2012) Amazon Digital Services LLC.

CLEAN WATER
Berkeyfilters.com (solid block carbon filter)
"Journey of Souls – Case Studies of Life between Lives" (2010) by Michael Newton, PhD.

"Destiny of Souls – Case Studies of Life between Lives" (2010) by Michael Newton, PhD.

"Many Lives, Many Masters: The True Story of a Prominent Psychiatrist, His Young Patient and The Past Life Therapy That changed both Their Lives" (2012) by Brian L. Weiss, MD.

"Through Life into Healing – Discovering the Power of Regression Therapy to erase Trauma and Transform Mind, Body and Relationships" (1992) by Brain L. Weiss, MD.

"The Twelve Stages of Healing – A Network Approach to Wholeness" (1994) by Donald M. Epstein, DC.

"Yoga as Medicine – The Yogic Prescription for Health and Healing" (2007) by Timothy McCall, MD, Bantam Books.

"Thriving After Breast Cancer – Essential Healing Exercises for Body and Mind" (2002) by Sherry Lebed Davis.

"Yoga For Cancer – Esoteric, Yogic & Dietary Remedies" (2010) by Bijoyalaxmi Hota.

"Effortless Mind – Meditate with Ease" by Ajayan Borys (2013) New World Library.

REFERENCES AND SOURCES

These deliberately do not appear in alphabetical order, but rather in the order they are referenced within each chapter.

CHAPTER TWO – WHY CANCER CAN GET A FOOTHOLD IN THE FIRST PLACE

https://www.cancer.gov/about-nci/legislative/history/national-cancer-act-1971#date

https://www.cdc.gov/nchs/data/hus/hus15.pdf#019

Bharti AC, Aggarwal BB "Nuclear factor-kappa B and cancer: its role in prevention and therapy". Biochem Pharmacol. 2002 Sep;64(5-6):883-8.

Aggarwal BB "Nuclear factor-kappa B: the enemy within". Cancer Cell. 2004 Sep;6(3):203-8.

Supic G, Jagodic M, Magic Z "Epigenetics: a new link between nutrition and cancer." Nutr. Cancer. 2013;65(6):781-92.

Carotenuto Felicia et al. "How Diet Intervention via Modulation of DNA Damage Response through MicroRNAs May Have an Effect on Cancer Prevention and Aging, an in Silico Study."

Ed. Guillermo T. Sáez. International Journal of Molecular Sciences 17.5 (2016): 752.

Bosutti Alessandra et al. "Epigenetic and miRNAs Dysregulation in Prostate Cancer: The Role of Nutraceuticals". Anti-Cancer Agents in Medicinal Chemistry 16.11 (2016): 1385–1402.

Bishop Karen S, Ferguson Lynnette R "The Interaction between Epigenetics, Nutrition and the Development of Cancer." Nutrients 7.2 (2015): 922–947.

Lee CH, Jeon YT, Kim SH, Song YS "NF-kappaB as a potential molecular target for cancer therapy". Biofactors. 2007;29(1):19-35.

Ichikawa H, Nakamura Y, Kashiwada Y, Aggarwal BB "Anticancer drugs designed by mother nature: ancient drugs but modern targets". Curr Pharm Des 2007; 13(33):3400-16

Kaefer CM, Milner J "The Role of Herbs and Spices in Cancer Prevention". J Nutr Biochem June 2008; 19(6):347-361.

Busch Christian et al. "Epigenetic Activities of Flavonoids in the Prevention and Treatment of Cancer." Clinical Epigenetics 7.1 (2015): 64.

Duggan Shane P, Gallagher William M, Fox Edward JP, Abdel-Latif Mohammed M, Reynolds John V, Kelleher D "Low pH induces co-ordinate regulation of gene expression in oesophageal cells." Carcinogenesis (Feb 2006) 27(2):319-327 first published online August 19, 2005.

Damaghi, Mehdi, Jonathan W. Wojtkowiak, and Robert J. Gillies.

"pH Sensing and Regulation in Cancer." Frontiers in Physiology 4 (2013): 370.

Kato, Yasumasa et al. "Acidic Extracellular Microenvironment and Cancer." Cancer Cell International 13 (2013): 89.

Surh YJ, Han SS, Keum YS, Seo HJ, Lee SS "Inhibitory effects of curcumin and capsaicin on phorbol ester-induced activation of eukaryotic transcription factors, NF-kappa B and AP-1." Biofactors. 2000:12(1-4):107-12.

Kewitz Stefanie, Volkmer Ines, Staege Martin S. "Curcuma Contra Cancer? Curcumin and Hodgkin's Lymphoma." Cancer Growth and Metastasis 6 (2013): 35-52.

Seyfried Thomas "Cancer as a Metabolic Disease: On the Origin, Management, and Prevention of Cancer". (2012) Wiley Publishing

Kremer Heinrich "The Silent Revolution in Cancer and AIDS Medicine". (2012) Xlibris Publishing

Coy Johannes F. Dr. Rer., Franz Maren "Die neue Anti-Krebs Ernährung – Wie Sie das Krebs Gen stoppen". (2009) Gräfe und Unzer Verlag

CHAPTER 3 – MAKE FOOD YOUR PERSONAL PHARMACY – HOW TO EAT SMART, NOT JUST RIGHT

Aggarwal BB, Van Kuiken ME, Sung B "Molecular targets of Neutraceuticals derived from dietary spices: Potential Role in Suppression of Inflammation & Tumorigenesis". Exp Biol Med (Maywood) 2009 Aug; 234(8):825-849.

Batty N, Malouf GG, Issa JP "Histone deacetylase inhibitors as anti-neoplastic agents". 2009 Aug, Cancer Letters 280(2):190-200.

Demetrakopoulos GE, Cancer Research, vol.42, p.756S, Feb.1982.

Gupta, Subash C. et al. "Regulation of Survival, Proliferation, Invasion, Angiogenesis, and Metastasis of Tumor Cells through Modulation of Inflammatory Pathways by Nutraceuticals." Cancer metastasis reviews 29.3 (2010): 405-434.

Gupta SC, Kim JH, Kannappan, R, Reuter S, Dougherty PM, Aggarwal BB "Role of NFKB-mediated inflammatory pathways in cancer-related symptoms & their regulation by nutritional agents". Exp Biol Med (Maywood) June 2011; 236(6):658-71.

IARC (WHO) GLOBOCAN 2012: "Estimated Cancer Incidence, Prevalence and Mortality Worldwide in 2012" http://globocan.iarc.fr/Pages/fact_sheets_cancer.aspx

Ho E, Dashwood RH "Dietary manipulation of histone structure & function". World Rev Nutr Diet. 2010; 101:95-102.

Ho V, Leung K, Hsu A, et.al. "A Low Carbohydrate, High Protein Diet Slows Tumor Growth and Prevents Cancer Initiation". Cancer Res 2011.

Kannappan R, Gupta SC, Aggarwal BB "Beuroprotection by spice-derived neutraceuticals: You are what you eat". Mol Neurobiol Oct 2011; 44(2):142-159.

Kim JH, Gupta SC, Aggarwal BB "Turmeric inhibits inflammatory NFKB". Mol Nutr Food Res March 2012; 56(3):454-465.

Laron Z "Insulin – A Growth Hormone". Arch Physiol Biochem. 2008 Feb; 114(1):11-6.

https://www.drweil.com/health-wellness/body-mind-spirit/disease-disorders/metabolic-syndrome/

ODPHP (Office of Disease Prevention and Health Promotion) of the US Department of Health and Human Services https://health.gov/

https://nutritiondata.self.com/

CDC National Center for Health Statistics https://www.cdc.gov/nchs/pressroom/

LeRoith D, Yakar S "Mechanisms of disease: metabolic effects of growth hormone and insulin-like growth factor 1". Nat Clin Pract Endocrinol Metab. 2007 Mar; 3(3): 302-10.

Zhang, Luoping et al. "Occupational Exposure to Formaldehyde, Hematotoxicity and Leukemia-Specific Chromosome Changes in Cultured Myeloid Progenitor Cells." Cancer epidemiology, biomarkers & prevention : a publication of the American Association for Cancer Research, cosponsored by the American Society of Preventive Oncology 19.1 (2010): 80–88. PMC. Web. 10 Mar. 2017.

Nielsen, Gunnar Damgård, Søren Thor Larsen, and Peder Wolkoff "Re-Evaluation of the WHO (2010) Formaldehyde Indoor Air Quality Guideline for Cancer Risk Assessment". Archives of Toxicology 91.1 (2017): 35–61. PMC. Web. 10 Mar. 2017.

Olney JW "Excitotoxins in foods." Neurotoxicology. 1994 Fall; 15(3):535-44.

Ibiebele TI, Nagle CM, Bain CJ, Webb PM "Intake of omega-3 and omega-6 fatty acids and risk of ovarian cancer". Cancer Causes Control. 2012 Nov;23(11):1775-83

https://www.healingjourneys.org/nutrition-and-cancer/ (Jeanne Wallace, PhD).

Myzak MC, Dashwood RH "Chemoprotection by sulforaphane: keep one eye beyond Keap1". Cancer Letter 2006; 233(2):208-218.

Prasad S, Ravindran J, Aggarwal BB "NFKB & Cancer: how intimate is this relationship?". Mol Cell Biochem March 2010; 336(1-2):25-37.

Ralhan R, Pandey MK, Aggarwal BB "NFKB links carcinogenic & chemopreventive agents". Front Biosci (School Ed) June 2009 1:1:45-60.

Sung B, Prasad S, Aggarwal BB "Cancer cell signaling pathways targeted by spice-derived neutraceuticals". Nutr Cancer 2012; 64(2):173-197.

CHAPTER 4 – REDUCING THE TOXIC EXPOSURE IN OUR FOOD SUPPLY

Labreche FP, Goldberg MS (1997). Exposure to organic solvents and breast cancer in women: A hypothesis". *Am J Ind Med,* 32:1-14. https://www.bcpp.org/resource/organic-solvents/

http://www.biography.com/people/rachel-carson-9239741#synopsis

http://www.rachelcarson.org/

Carson Rachel "Silent Spring" (1962), Houghton Mifflin Company

http://www.nytimes.com/2012/09/23/magazine/how-silent-spring-ignited-the-environmental-movement.html

https://en.wikipedia.org/wiki/Rachel_Carson

https://www.epa.gov/ingredients-used-pesticide-products/ddt-brief-history-and-status

https://en.wikipedia.org/wiki/Pesticide_regulation_in_the_United_States

Randolph G. Theron, MD, Moss Ralph M. PhD. " An Alternative Approach to Allergies – The New Field of Clinical Ecology Unravels the Environmental Causes of Mental and Physical Ills", Revised Edition (1990), William Morrow Paperbacks

Francis Raymond MSc "Never Fear Cancer Again: How to Prevent and Reverse Cancer" (2011) HCI Publisher, 1st edition

2008-2009 President's Cancer Panel Report:
https://deainfo.nci.nih.gov/advisory/pcp/annualreports/pcp08-09rpt/pcp_report_08-09_508.pdf

https://www.cdc.gov/biomonitoring/pdf/FourthReport_

UpdatedTables_Volume1_Jan2017.pdf

https://www.cdc.gov/exposurereport/

Testimony of Kenneth A. Cook President Environmental Working Group Before the SUBCOMMITTEE ON SUPERFUND, TOXICS AND ENVIRONMENTAL HEALTH U.S. SENATE COMMITTEEE ON ENVIRONMENT & PUBLIC WORKS On "Current Science on Public Exposures to Toxic Chemicals" Thursday, February 4, 2010 https://www.epw.senate.gov/public/_cache/files/31bcb6cf-26ff-4415-b04d-87988118af33/kencooktestimony0204100.pdf

EWG: Toxins found in umbilical cords of newborns http://www.ewg.org/news/news-releases/2009/02/18/ewg-asks-epa-chief-support-toxics-reform-bill

Role of FDA
https://www.fda.gov/AboutFDA/WhatWeDo/

GRAS status categorization
https://www.fda.gov/Food/IngredientsPackagingLabeling/GRAS/

Role of EPA
https://www.epa.gov/aboutepa/our-mission-and-what-we-do

Role of USDA (FSIS)
https://www.fsis.usda.gov/wps/portal/informational/aboutfsis/about-us

Dessey Mira NE "The Pantry Principle – How to read the label and understand what's really in your food" (2013) Versadia Press

Sacks Stephanie "What the Fork are you Eating? An Action Plan for Your Pantry and Plate" (2014) Tarcher Perigree Publisher (Penguin Group), 1st edition

Mamur S, Yüzbaiolu D, Unal F, Yilmaz S "Does potassium sorbate induce genotoxic or mutagenic effects in lymphocytes?" Toxicol In Vitro. 2010;24:790-4.

Kitano K, Fukukawa T, Ohtsuji Y, Masuda T, Yamaguchi H "Mutagenicity and DNA-damaging activity caused by decomposed products of potassium sorbate reacting with ascorbic acid in the presence of Fe salt". Food Chem Toxicol. 2002;40:1589-94.

Hauter Wenonah, Worth Mark "Zapped! Irradiation and the Death of Food" (2008) Food and Water Watch Press

Questions and Answers on MSG (answered by the FDA)
https://www.fda.gov/Food/IngredientsPackagingLabeling/
FoodAdditivesIngredients/ucm328728.htm
Report by CSPI (2010) on Food Dyes: A Rainbow of Risks
https://cspinet.org/resource/food-dyes-rainbow-risks

Comments made by Michael F. Jacobsen, Executive Director of the CSPI and James Huff, Associate at the National Toxicology Program

Food Dyes linked to Cancer, ADHA and Allergies http://www.
foodsafetynews.com/2010/07/popular-food-dyes-linked-to-
cancer-adhd-and-allergies/
http://sitn.hms.harvard.edu/flash/2015/gmos-and-pesticides/

Re-evaluation of food colours: EFSA completes major programme (2016)
http://www.efsa.europa.eu/en/press/news/160914a

EU Food Information to Consumers legislation
http://ec.europa.eu/food/safety/labelling_nutrition/labelling_legislation_en

EU places warning labels on foods containing dyes (2010)
http://www.foodsafetynews.com/2010/07/eu-places-warning-labels-on-foods-containing-dyes/

Potera Carol "Diet and Nutrition: The Artificial Food Dye Blues".
Environ. Health Perspect 118:a428(2010).

The Pursuit of Sweet article on Saccharin
https://www.chemheritage.org/distillations/magazine/the-pursuit-of-sweet

Saccharin Study and Labeling Act of 1977
https://www.govtrack.us/congress/bills/95/s1750
https://en.wikipedia.org/wiki/Saccharin_Study_and_Labeling_Act_of_1977

Splenda leading to a depletion of healthy gut bacteria
Nestle, Marion "Safe Food – The Politics of Food Safety" (2010),
University of California Press.

https://www.scientificamerican.com/article/artificial-sweeteners-may-change-our-gut-bacteria-in-dangerous-ways/

Aspartame and cancer risk

http://articles.mercola.com/sites/articles/archive/2011/10/15/this-artificial-sweetener-shown-to-produce-cancer-in-rats.aspx

Dangers of chlorine
http://articles.mercola.com/sites/articles/archive/2001/06/23/chlorine-part-two.aspx

The NON-GMO Project
https://www.nongmoproject.org/about/

Agave Nectar as an alternative sweetener
https://www.drweil.com/diet-nutrition/nutrition/whats-wrong-with-agave-nectar/

https://draxe.com/agave-nectar/

Coca-Cola sued, others settle cases over cancer-causing benzene8/25/2006
http://usatoday30.usatoday.com/money/industries/food/2006-08-25-coke-benzene_x.htm

2006 Harvard Study on Trans Fats
https://www.hsph.harvard.edu/nutritionsource/transfats/

FDA labeling requirements for Trans Fats
https://askfsis.custhelp.com/app/answers/detail/a_id/1324/~/fda%E2%80%99s-requirements-for-nutrition-labeling-of-trans-fats

Alavanja MCR. "Pesticides Use and Exposure Extensive Worldwide. Reviews on environmental health". 2009;24(4):303-309.

USDA Pesticide Data Program
https://www.ams.usda.gov/datasets/pdp

Pesticide Data Program Annual Summary 2015
https://www.ams.usda.gov/sites/default/files/media/2015PD-PAnnualSummary.pdf

Monsanto guilty of chemical poisoning in France http://www.reuters.com/article/us-france-pesticides-monsanto-idUS-TRE81C0VQ20120213

Monsanto suing small farms to protect seed patents https://www.theguardian.com/environment/2013/feb/12/monsanto-sues-farmers-seed-patents

EWGs Shopper's Guide to Pesticides in Produce
https://www.ewg.org/foodnews/summary.php

Food Inc. Movie
http://www.imdb.com/title/tt1286537/

Facts on Antibiotic Use
http://www.foodsafetynews.com/2011/02/fda-confirms-80-percent-of-antibiotics-used-in-animal-ag/

Antibiotic use in livestock
https://www.nytimes.com/2014/10/03/science/antibiotics-in-livestock-fda-finds-use-is-rising.html?_r=0

AWA
https://www.awanj.org/

Certified Humane
http://certifiedhumane.org/

Local Harvest
http://www.localharvest.org

FDA on approval of use of hormones
https://www.fda.gov/AnimalVeterinary/SafetyHealth/Prod-uctSafetyInformation/ucm055436.htm

EU on use of hormones in meat
https://ec.europa.eu/food/safety/chemical_safety/meat_hor-mones_en

About genetically engineered foods
http://www.centerforfoodsafety.org/issues/311/ge-foods/about-ge-foods

On Glyphosate
http://npic.orst.edu/factsheets/glyphogen.html
http://drpompa.com/additional-resources/health-tips/the-dangers-of-glyphosate-an-interview-with-dr-stephanie-seneff

Defarge N, Takács E, Lozano VL, Mesnage R, Spiroux de Vendômois J, Séralini GE, Székács A "Co_formulants in Glyphosate-Based Herbicides Disrupt Aromatase Activity in Human Cells below Toxic Levels". Int J Environ Res Public Health. 2016 Feb26;13(3).

Bøhn T, Cuhra M, Traavik T, Sanden M, Fagan J, Primicerio R "Compositional Differences in soybeans on the market: glyphosate accumulates in Roundup Ready GM soybeans". Food Chem.

2014 Jun15;153:207-15.

Thongprakaisang S, Thiantanawat A, Rangkadilok N, Suriyo T, Satayavivad J "Glyphosate induces human breast cancer cell growth via estrogen receptors", Food Chem Toxicol. 2013 Sep;59:129-36.

Dr. Dean Burk, *Congressional Record 21 July 1976*
Dr Dean Burk Interview   https://www.youtube.com/watch?v=kzgKA5zMitQ

Fluoridation http://www.rethinkingcancer.org/resources/magazine-articles/2_3-4/fluoridation.php

http://fluoridealert.org/content/top_ten/

https://thetruthaboutcancer.com/fluoride-drinking-our-selves-to-death/

http://fluoridealert.org/researchers/fda/not-approved/

The Frank R. Lautenberg Chemical Safety for the 21st Century Act https://www.epa.gov/assessing-and-managing-chemicals-under-tsca/frank-r-lautenberg-chemical-safety-21st-century-act-0#pbt

EPA's Home Drinking Water Filtration Fact Sheet: https://www.epa.gov/ground-water-and-drinking-water/home-drinking-water-filtration-fact-sheet

http://www.ro-system.org/

http://waterfilters.mercola.com/drinking-water-filter.aspx
http://www.berkeyfilters.com

CHAPTER 5 – REDUCING THE TOXIC EXPOSURE IN OUR HOMES

Epstein Samuel, PhD, Steinman David "The Safe Shopper's Bible – A Consumer's Guide to Nontoxic Household Products, Cosmetics and Food" (1995), Wiley Publishers

Chemicals in Cosmetics (Breast Cancer Prevention Partners – BCPP)
https://www.bcpp.org/?s=chemicals+in+cosmetics

EWG's Skin Deep Cosmetics Database
http://www.ewg.org/skindeep/

The danger with Sodium Lauryl Sulfates
http://articles.mercola.com/sites/articles/archive/2010/07/13/sodium-lauryl-sulfate.aspx

NCI on dangers of Formaldehyde (NCI)
https://www.cancer.gov/about-cancer/causes-prevention/risk/substances/formaldehyde/formaldehyde-fact-sheet

IARC classifies formaldehyde as a carcinogen
https://www.iarc.fr/en/media-centre/pr/2004/pr153.html

National Toxicology Report, 14th edition, on Formaldehyde as a carcinogen
https://ntp.niehs.nih.gov/ntp/roc/content/profiles/formaldehyde.pdf

EWG's Guide to Healthy Cleaning
http://www.ewg.org/guides/cleaners/content/cleaners_and_
health

Electromagnetic Fields and Public Health (WHO report)
http://www.who.int/peh-emf/publications/facts/fs296/en/

Burk Larry M.D. "Let Magic Happen – Adventures in healing
with a Holistic Radiologist" (2012) Healing Imager Press

Dr Debra Davis and the Environmental Health Trust
http://ehtrust.org/about/dr-devra-davis/

Davis Debra "Disconnect: The Truth About Cell Phone Radiation,
What the Industry is Doing to Hide It, and How To Protect Your
Family" (2011), Plume Publisher

IARC Report on RF-EMF as Group 2B carcinogens
http://www.iarc.fr/en/media-centre/pr/2011/pdfs/pr208_E.
pdf

Ober Clinto, Sinatra Stephen T. M.D. "Earthing: The Most
Important Health Discovery Ever!"(2014), Basic Health Publications, Inc.

Hetherington Michael "Getting Grounded: For Health and Healing" (2015) Amazon Digital Services LLC

Does your cell phone case raise radiation exposure
http://www.ewg.org/research/does-your-cell-phone-case-
raise-your-radiation-exposure

Dr Ibrahim Karim and BioGeometry
https://www.biogeometry.ca/home

International Institute for Bau-biologie and Ecology
http://www.gbb.org/business/international-institute-for-bau-biologie-ecology/

Wireless acts synergistically with toxic exposure to significantly increase cancer risk
http://ehtrust.org/key-issues/the-environment-and-health/wireless-radiationelectromagnetic-fields-increases-toxic-body-burden/

Labreche FP, Goldberg MS "Exposure to organic solvents and breast cancer in women: A hypothesis". Am J Ind Med, 1997, 32:1-14.

Halgamuge MN, "Pineal melatonin level disruption in humans due to electromagnetic fields and ICNIRP limits". Radiat Prot Dosimetry. 2013 May;154(4):405-16.

Gultekin David H, Moeller Lothar "NMR Imaging of Cell Phone Radiation Absorption in Brain Tissue." Proceedings of the National Academy of Sciences of the United States of America 110.1 (2013): 58–63. *PMC*. Web. 12 Feb. 2017.

Cardis E, Varsier N, Bowman JD, Deltour I, Figuerola J, Mann S, Moissonnier M, Taki M, Vecchia P, Villegas R, Vrijheid M, Wake K, Wiart J "Estimation of RF energy absorbed in the brain from mobile phones in the Interphone Study". Occup Environ Med. 2011 Sep;68(9):686-93.

CHAPTER 6 – USE YOUR CONSCIOUS MIND

Shapiro Deb "Your Body Speaks Your Mind – Understanding How Your Emotions and Thoughts Affect You Physically" (1996) Piatkus Books.

Illibagiza Immaculaeé "Left to tell – Discovering God Amidst the Rwandan Holocaust" (2013) Hay House Publishing.

Emoto Masaru Dr. "The Healing Power of Water" (2008) Hay House Publishing.

Lipton Bruce H, PhD "The Biology of Belief: Unleashing the Power of Consciousness, matter and Miracles" (2005), Bruce H. Lipton, Mountain of Love Productions Inc. and Elite Books, San Rafael, CA.

https://www.brucelipton.com/

Dispenza Joe Dr. "Breaking the Habit of Being Yourself – How to Lose Your Mind and Create an New One" (2012) Hay House Publishing.

https://www.drjoedispenza.com/
https://plato.stanford.edu/entries/descartes-works/

http://www.biography.com/people/ren-descartes-37613#synopsis

http://www.biography.com/people/isaac-newton-9422656

http://www.history.com/topics/isaac-newton

http://www.history.com/this-day-in-history/the-birth-of-quantum-theory

http://www.informationphilosopher.com/quantum/history

Purves D, Augustine GJ, Fitzpatrick D, et al., "Physiological changes associated with emotion" Neuroscience 2nd edition, Sunderland (MA): Sinauer Associates; 2001.

McCraty Rollin, Atkinson Mike, and Tomasino Dana "Modulation of DNA conformation by heart-focused intention." Heart-Math Research Center, Institute of HeartMath, Publication No. 03-008. Boulder Creek, CA (2003): 2.

Bowder Will "A Complaint Free World – How to Stop Complaining and Start Enjoying the Life You Always Wanted" (2007) Doubleday Publishing

CHAPTER 7 ALLOW EMOTIONAL HEALING

Weiss Brian L. M.D. "Through Time into Healing – Discovering the Power of Regression Therapy to Erase Trauma and Transform Mind, Body and Relationships" (1993), Touchstone Publisher.

De Wet Pieter M.D. "Heal Thyself – Transform Your Life Transform Your Health" (2010) Tate Publishing & Enterprises.

Nelson Bradley, M.D. "The Emotion Code – How to Release Your Trapped Emotions for Abundant Health, Love and Happiness" (2007) Wellness Unmasked Publishing.

Monti DA, Stoner ME, Zivin G, Schlesinger M "Short term correlates of the Neuro Emotional Technique for cancer-related traumatic stress symptoms: a pilot case series". J Cancer Surviv. 2007 Jun;1(2):161-6.

Monti DA, Tobia A, Stoner M, Wintering N, Matthews M, He XS, Doucet G, Chervoneva I, Tracy JI, Newberg AB "Neuro Emotional Technique effects on brain physiology in cancer patients with traumatic stress symptoms: preliminary findings". J Cancer Surviv. 2017 Feb 8.

https://www.netmindbody.com/for-patients/an-explana-tion-of-net

McLay Robert N, Webb-Murphy Jennifer A, Fesperman Susan F, Delaney Eileen M, Gerard Steven K, Roesch Scott C, Nebeker Bonnie J, Pandzic Ines, Vishnyak Elizabeth A, Johnston Scott L "Outcomes from eye movement desensitization and reprocess-ing in active-duty service members with posttraumatic stress disorder". Psychological Trauma: Theory, Research, Practice, and Policy, Vol 8(6), Nov 2016, 702-708.

Gerhardt Andreas et al. "Eye Movement Desensitization and Reprocessing vs. Treatment-as-Usual for Non-Specific Chronic Back Pain Patients with Psychological Trauma: A Randomized Controlled Pilot Study". Frontiers in Psychiatry. 2016; 7: 201.

Bossini L, Casolaro I, Santarnecchi E, Caterini C, Koukouna D, Fernandez I, Fagiolini A "Evaluation Study of clinical and neuro-biological efficacy of EMDR in patients suffering from post-trau-matic stress disorder". Riv Psichiatr. 2012 Mar-Apr;47(2 Suppl):12-5.

http://www.emdr.com/

Shapiro Francine, "Getting Past your Past: Take Control of Your Life with Self-Help Techniques from EMDR Therapy" (2013) Rodale Books.

http://www.reiki.org/

Cheek David, LeCron Leslie, "Clinical Hypnotherapy" (1968) Grune & Stratton.
Detzler Robert "The Freedom Path" (2006) Spiritual Response Center.

https://spiritualresponse.com/

The Association for Applied Psychophysiology and Biofeedback
http://www.aapb.org/i4a/pages/index.cfm?pageid=1

http://www.emofree.com/

http://www.acos.org/articles/the-chinese-medicine-meridian-system/

http://www.thetappingsolution.com/what-is-eft-tapping/

http://eft.mercola.com/

https://wiseworldseminars.com/network-spinal-analysis

Epstein Donald M, D.C. "The Twelve Stages of Healing – A Network Approach to Wholeness" (1994) Amber Allen Publishing.

CHAPTER 8 – GET MOVING CHAPTER

Dimeo F, Stieglitz RD, Novelli-Fischer U et al. "Effects of aerobic exercise on fatigue and psychological status of cancer patients during chemotherapy". Cancer 1998; 85: 2273-7

Christensen JF, Jones LW, Andersen JL, Daugaard G, Rorth M, Hojman P "Muscle dysfunction in cancer patients". Ann Oncol 2014; 25 (5): 947-958.
Al-Majid S, McCarthy DO "Cancer-induced fatigue and skeletal muscle wasting: the role of exericise". Biological Research for Nursing. 2(3):186-97, 2001.

Baracos, VE "Management of muscle wasting in cancer-associated cachexia". Cancer, 2001. 92: 1669–1677.

Meyerhardt JA, Heseltine D, Niedzwiecki D, Hollis D, Saltz LB, Mayer RJ, Thomas J, Nelson H, Whittom R, Hantel A, Schilsky RL, Fuchs CS. „Impact of Physical activity on cancer recurrence and survival in patients with stage III colon cancer: findings from CALGB 89803". J Clin Oncol. 2006 Aug 1;24(22):3535-41.

Holmes MD, Chen WY, Feskanich D, Kroenke CH, Colditz GA "Physical activity and survival after breast cancer diagnosis". JAMA. 2005 May 25;293(20):2479-86.

Lahart IM, Metsios GS, Nevill AM, Carmichael AR "Physical activity, risk of death and recurrence in breast cancer survivors: A systematic review and meta-analysis of epidemiological studies". Acta. Oncol. 2015 May;54(5):635-54

Block Keith M.D. "Life Over Cancer – The Block Center Program for Integrative Cancer Treatment" (2009) Bantam Books.

Mormont MC, Waterhouse J, Bleuzen P, Giacchetti S, Jami A, Bogdan A, Lellouch J, Misset JL, Touitou Y, Lévi F "Marked 24-h rest/activity rhythms are associated with better quality of life, better response, and longer survival in patients with metastatic colorectal cancer and good performance status". Clin Cancer Res. 2000 Aug;6(8):3038-45.

Fairey AS, Courneya KS, Field CJ, Bell GJ, Jones LW, Mackey JR "Effects of exercise training on fasting insulin, insulin resistance, insulin-like growth factors, and insulin-like growth factor binding proteins in postmenopausal breast cancer survivors: a randomized controlled trial". Cancer Epidemiol Biomarkers Prev. 2003 Aug;12(8):721-7.

Bigley AB, Simpson RJ "NK cells and exercise: implications for cancer immunotherapy and survivorship". Discov Med. 2015 Jun;19(107):433-45.

Circadian Rhythm Fact Sheet
https://publications.nigms.nih.gov/syndication/factsheet_circadianrhythms.htm

Savvidis C, & Koutsilieris M, (2012). "Circadian Rhythm Disruption in Cancer Biology". Molecular Medicine, 18(1), 1249–1260.

IARC Working Group on the Evaluation of Carcinogenic Risks to Humans. (2010). "Painting, firefighting, and shiftwork. IARC Monographs on the Evaluation of Carcinogenic Risks to Humans", 98, 9–764.

https://sleepfoundation.org/sleep-topics/sleep-drive-and-your-body-clock

http://www.health.harvard.edu/staying-healthy/take-a-deep-breath

Conrad A, Müller A, Doberenz S, Kim S, Meuret AE, Wollburg E, Roth WT "Psychophysiological effects of breathing instructions for stress management". Appl Psychophysiol Biofeedback. 2007 Jun;32(2):89-98.

Han, JN, et al. "Unsteadiness of breathing in patients with hyperventilation syndrome and anxiety disorders". European Respiratory Journal 10.1 (1997): 167-176.

https://www.cancer.org/treatment/treatments-and-side-effects/physical-side-effects/shortness-of-breath.html

Abdou AM, Higashiguchi S, Horie K, Kim M, Hatta H, Yokogoshi H "Relaxation and immunity enhancement effects of gamma-aminobutyric acid (GABA) administration in humans". Biofactors. 2006;26(3):201-8.

Rebounder
https://en.wikipedia.org/wiki/Rebound_exercise

Sagar SM, M.D., Dryden T, Med RMT, Wong RK, M.D. "Massage therapy for cancer patients: a reciprocal relationship between body and mind". Curr Oncol. 2007 Apr; 14(2): 45-56

Cranio-Sacraltherapy: http://www.upledger.com/about/index.php

The Global BMI Mortality Collaboration. "Body-mass index and all-cause mortality: individual-participant-data meta-analysis of 239 prospective studies in four continents". Lancet (2016) (London, England), 388(10046), 776–786. http://doi.org/10.1016/S0140-6736(16)30175-1

Tomiyama AJ, Hunger JM, Mguyen-Cuu J, Wells C "Misclassification of cardiometabolic health when using body mass index categories in NHANES 2005-2012". Int J Obes (Lond). 2016 May;40(5):883-6.

Smart BMI Calculator
http://www.smartbmicalculator.com/why-sbmic.html

Bailor Jonathan "The Calorie Myth: How to Eat More, Exercise Less, Lose Weight and Live Better" (2015) Harper Wave Publishing.

Leinhart Peter, Seibert Wolfgang "Funktionelles Bewegungstraining – Muskuläre Dysbalance erkennen, beseitigen und vermeiden" (2001), 6. Auflage, Urban & Fischer Verlag.

About the Author

Kirstin is an empathetic cancer mentor, speaker and educator, who is passionate about enabling anyone associated with cancer to pro-actively and holistically navigate their health challenge. After being diagnosed with breast cancer twice within three years, she learnt first-hand the importance of an integrative and functional medicine approach to one's health, acknowledging the dynamic interdependency of body, mind and soul to facilitate true healing.

Kirstin is the founder of Eat Holistic LLC and offers individualized 1 on 1 mentoring, can be hired for inspirational speaking engagements and produces interactive virtual programs such as the Beyond Cancer Program™.

She is a co-host for the #AllThingsCancer podcast, a monthly guest-blogger for The Anti-Cancer Club, has frequently featured in a variety of holistic Internet Radio Shows and online Podcasts and was a monthly contributing author for the online Sybil Magazine – For the Spirit and Soul of Woman.

Born in Switzerland, raised in Germany and South Africa, she now lives in NJ with her husband, adult son, teenage daughter and spunky Wirehaired Pointer Max.

Connect with Kirstin

1. PERSONALIZED MENTORING SESSIONS

If you are ready to take your cancer journey to the next level, connect with Kirstin to book a free 15-minute Assessment Session where you and Kirstin can get to know each other a little and decide if you are a good fit. Book your session here.

2. INTERACTIVE ONLINE PROGRAMS

If you would like to educate yourself in the comfort of your own home, and allow me to teach you how you can take pro-active steps to conquer cancer and reclaim your health, join me on one of my virtual, online programs. Click here to read more.

3. HIRE KIRSTIN AS A KEYNOTE SPEAKER FOR YOUR EVENT

I am passionate about empowering your audience to make informed and evidence-based decisions when it comes to an integratve approach to cancer care. Click here to find out more on my Press page

Website:
www.kirstinscancercare.com
Email:
kirstin@kirstinscancercare.com

Feel free to follow Kirstin on Facebook at
https://www.facebook.com/kirstinscancercare/

Connect on Twitter
https://twitter.com/

Connect on LinkedIn
https://www.linkedin.com/in/kirstin-nussgruber-911b0643/

Kirstin's Amazon Author Page
https://authorcentral.amazon.com/gp/profile

ONE LAST THING…

If you enjoyed this book or found it useful I'd be very grateful if you'd post a short review on Amazon. Your support really does make a difference and I read all the reviews personally to improve how I serve the cancer-thriver community.

If you'd like to leave a review then all you need to do is click the review link on this book's page on Amazon, or find it by clicking right here.

http://amzn.to/2qEOdKb

Thank you very much again for your support!

With deep appreciation

Made in the USA
Middletown, DE
13 July 2017